CW01471812

# Drop a
# dress size

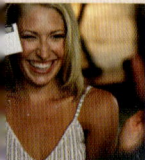

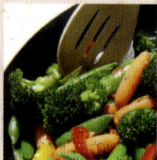

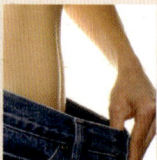

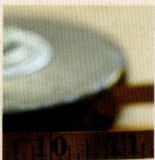

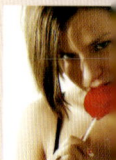

# Drop a
# dress size

52 brilliant little ideas to
lose weight and stay slim

## Eve Cameron and Kate Cook

brilliant ideas

## CAREFUL NOW

Follow the tips in this book and you should find that you not only lose weight but also keep that weight off. The key to staying slim is losing the weight slowly and changing your habits, so don't expect instant results. Be careful: don't be too ambitious about how much weight you want to lose or how quickly you want to do it and consult your GP before embarking on a radical new diet or exercise plan or taking any supplements. We wish you every success – good luck!

Infinite Ideas would like to thank Linda Bird, Eve Cameron, Steve Shipside and Kate Cook for their contributions to this book.

Copyright © The Infinite Ideas Company Ltd, 2006

The right of the contributors to be identified as the authors of this book has been asserted in accordance with the Copyright, Designs and Patents Act 1988.

First published in 2006 by
**The Infinite Ideas Company Limited**
36 St Giles
Oxford, OX1 3LD
United Kingdom
www.infideas.com

Reprinted 2007

A CIP catalogue record for this book is available from the British Library
ISBN 978-1-904902-06-5

Brand and product names are trademarks or registered trademarks of their respective owners.

Designed and typeset by Baseline Arts Ltd, Oxford
Printed in China

# Brilliant ideas

# Introduction

**How do I get the body I want, so I can fit
into the clothes I love?**

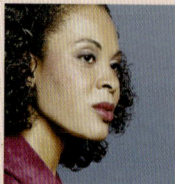

If you're loking for a diet book that succeeds
where others have failed then look no further. The simple ideas in
this book won't take you hours to read and are just as quick and
easy to implement.

With its bite-sized ideas that cut the waffle and get straight down to
what you want to know we hope you'll find this book refreshingly
different. This is a more holistic guide to losing weight than
conventional dieting books. It deals with motivation, body shape,
healthy eating, decoding food labels, fitness and examines popular
diets and much more! It also introduces the idea that weight loss is
part of an over all healthy eating and lifestyle plan that will not only
make you slimmer but also put a spring in your step and give you
more energy for life.

Throughout the book, you'll find some recurring themes, which we
think are the key facets of successful weight loss:

■ *Diets are not something to be jumped on and off like buses.* The only way to lose weight permanently is to change your eating habits for good. Small changes and a long-term view are more successful than short-term bursts of enthusiasm.

■ *Physical activity is a must.* That doesn't mean working out at the gym every night of the week. But what it does mean is getting at least half an hour's moderate exercise five times a week. If you can find something you enjoy doing that also helps you slim down then you're more likely to stick at it.

■ *Realistic goals are essential for motivation and success.* You cannot change your basic body shape, all you can do is reduce the amount of fat you have and tone up your muscles. If you set yourself achievable targets you'll get there. Goals that are impossible to reach just make you miserable. Slow and steady is much better than a crash diet and you're more likely to keep the weight off.

■ *Learn to cook.* It takes the same amount of time to whip up a tasty, healthy, weight-loss-friendly meal as it does to reheat a ready meal or get a takeaway. The price isn't that different either. The only difference is to your waistline.

This book gives you all the knowledge, tips and ideas you'll need in small portions that will get you to where you want to be. So why not start today.

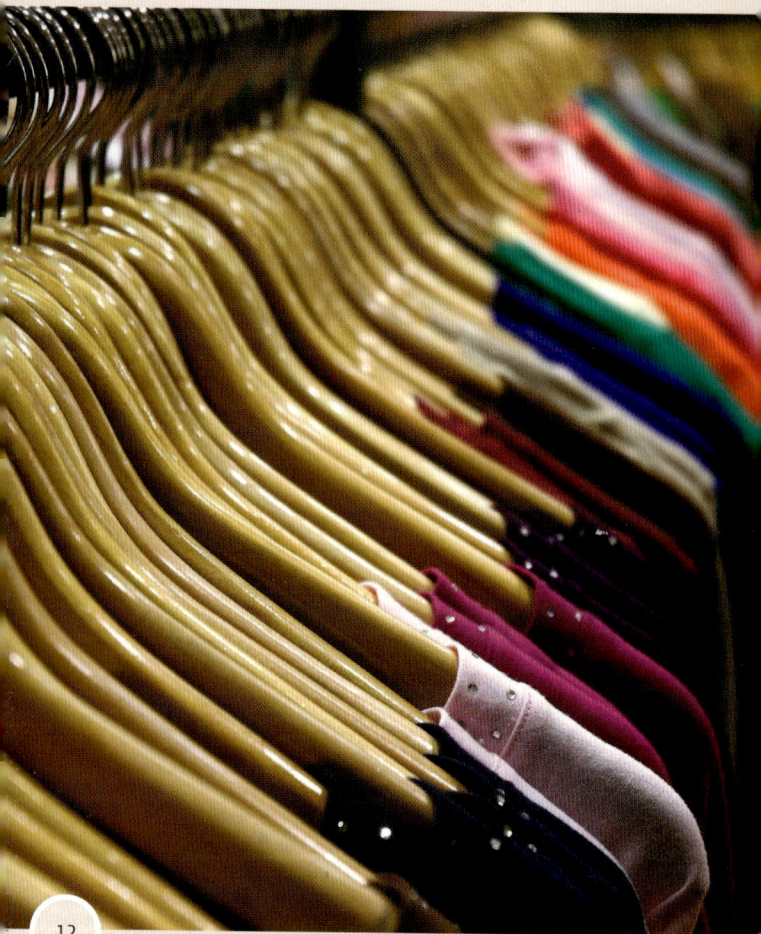

# 1. Why it's hard to lose weight

**Weight loss is for life and not just for after Christmas**

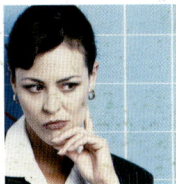

Instead of a short-term diet, find a way to eat for life that works yet doesn't make you feel like you're depriving yourself. The trouble with most diets is that too much organisation, time, concentration and effort is required to count calories or portion sizes. And let's face it; if diets worked the diet industry wouldn't be worth millions. Diets mean that we're thinking about food the whole time, so naturally we eat more or crack under the pressure of it all and have ten chocolate bars in one hit. Of course, if you eat a tub of lard every day then you might put on weight. Part of the equation of weight gain is calories in versus calories expended, but this is only part of the jigsaw. Think of all those people who eat exactly what and when they want and never put on an ounce. This proves that something else must be at work.

This something else isn't just one factor, but many. Gut health (including elimination), the level of

### Defining idea

'Physical fitness isn't only one of the most important keys to a healthy body, it is also the basis of dynamic and creative intellectual activity.'
**JOHN F. KENNEDY**

## Here's an idea for you...

If you're really determined to lose weight, why not really focus on it for a week? Start as you mean to go on and bin unhealthy packages lurking in your cupboards and fridge. Then get hold of the right ingredients: fresh foods and basic dry ingredients like lentils, chickpeas and brown rice, and nuts, seeds and dried fruit, which are good for snacks.

yeast in your system, how your immune system is functioning and your hormonal health (including that of your thyroid) can all have an effect on your metabolism and how you'll process the food you're eating. Of course, it may be that you're eating all the wrong foods and too much of them, but it might be something else as well. This book should give you some ideas.

The bad news is that change is often hard work because it requires you to do something differently. It's that old-fashioned word 'discipline' that freaks people out, but it simply means sticking to a healthy eating plan most of the time, which means when the mood strikes you, you can go crazy.

Nearly forgot. Best to get some exercise in too! Apart from the obvious thermodynamic reasons, exercise helps the metabolic functions – breathing, digestion and circulation – to work better. It's like having a powerful car – don't let it rust up in the garage, you need to take it for a spin. Give your body the right fuel and it will run beautifully.

# 2. A weighty issue

**Here's how to work out roughly the right weight for you, plus some news you can use about body shape.**

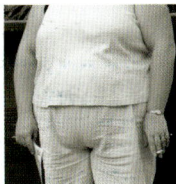

Judging by the newspaper headlines screaming about some new statistic or research about obesity, you'd think there was a moral obligation to be thin. Often the subtext is that fat people get sick and are a burden on our medical resources. And then there are the images of super-slim models and celebrities that confront us in magazines and on our TV and movie screens. The underlying message here is that this is the way you're supposed to look, especially if you want to be happy and successful, not to mention being sexually attractive.

But how overweight do you have to be before you have a problem? Working out if you're really overweight is easily done using the Body Mass Index calculation. I have to point out that this method is not

*Defining idea*

'I'm not overweight. I'm just nine inches too short.'
**SHELLEY WINTERS**

without its critics (partly because if you're quite well-muscled, you'll be heavy, not fat, because muscle weighs more than fat) but my feeling is you have to start somewhere! All you have to do is weigh

## Here's an idea for you...

Measure your waist and hips. Many experts are now saying that abdominal fat is the killer, with apple-shaped people who have relatively slim hips and a larger waist being more at risk from developing heart disease than the pear-shaped – those who carry their fat on their hips and thighs. The ideal waist measurement for men is less than 95 cm (37 inches) and less than 80 cm (32 inches) for women. Over 100 cm (40 inches) for a man and over 90 cm (35 inches) for a woman indicates the greatest risk to health.

yourself and record the result in kilograms. Then measure your height in metres. Then do the following sum:

weight in kilograms divided by (height in metres × height in metres) = BMI

Example:
You weigh 70 kg and you are 1.6 metres tall
$70 \div (1.6 \times 1.6) =$
$70 \div 2.56 = 27.34$
BMI = 27.34

Check your own result against the ranges below

| BMI for men | BMI for women | |
|---|---|---|
| Under 20 | under 19 | underweight |
| 20–24.9 | 19–24.9 | normal |
| 25–29.9 | 25–29.9 | overweight |
| 30 plus | 30 plus | obese |

I fall into the upper level of normal weight, which is fine from a fatness perspective, but I know that I've crept up two dress sizes in the past decade and so estimate that losing three kilos (and keeping it off!) would take me where I want to be. That's my weight-loss mission; now work out yours.

# 3. Food accountancy made simple

**Here's why knowing your calories is the key to losing weight**

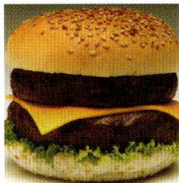

Many books make calories unnecessarily hard to understand, but the concept is really quite simple. Calories are just the basic units by which both the energy values of food and the energy needs of the body are measured. You may be familiar with diets that advocate counting your daily calorie intake. It's now seen as a rather old-fashioned way to slim, not least because you have to weigh things obsessively and eating anywhere but at home becomes a nightmare. However it is really important to have some idea of how many calories will make you gain weight.

Here's an idea for you...

Include soya products in your diet. A particular isoflavone in soya may hold the key to improving the rate at which your cells burn up fat. It also boosts your metabolism slightly and reduces your appetite. From a looks perspective, I have it on good authority that soya helps to make your nails grow too!

## How many calories do you need?

Here's a basic formula to work this out (calculators at the ready!); it will only be an approximate calculation but should still be enlightening:

First work out your *basal metabolic rate* (BMR) which tells you the energy you need to stay alive. Multiply your weight in pounds by 10 if you're a woman, or 11 if you're a man. (If you're a metric sort of person, first multiply your weight in kilos by 2.2 to get the poundage.) Next, factor in how active you are by multiplying the sum above by 0.2 if you only do very light activities, by 0.3 if you do a little more formal exercise such as walking as well as housework, by 0.4 if you are moderately active and you rarely sit still or by 0.5 if your job involves manual labour or you play lots of sports. The result is the number of calories you need on top of your BMR.

Eating and digesting food uses up around 10% of your calorie needs, so, after adding your BMR and the extra calories you worked out for your activity levels together, work out what 10% is. Now add all three of those figures together and you'll have the number of your total calorie needs per day.

To lose half a kilo (a pound) a week, you need to cut your daily calories by 500 (or cut fewer than that and make up the difference with exercise), which is a safe amount to aim for. Although this might not sound a lot, it's easier to achieve in the long term and easier to sustain. If you lose lots of weight very quickly, you're more likely to put it back on and get into that yo-yo dieting spiral.

OK, end of accountancy lesson.

## *Defining idea*

*'Two out of every three men in the UK are now classed as overweight or obese.'*
**THE BRITISH DIETETIC ASSOCIATION**

# 4. Setting goals

**Master the art of goal-setting to turn your dream of losing weight into reality. Planning really works!**

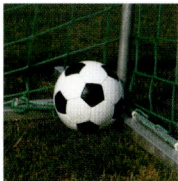

A well-known study of a group of US students in the 1950s found that only 3% of the graduates wrote a set of goals for their lives. A follow-up survey some twenty years later discovered that the goal-setting students were worth more financially than the other 97% put together; they were also healthier and happier in their relationships than the others.

Setting goals is a major step in slimming successfully. You can take it further by developing it like a formal business plan.

Goals need to be SMART: that's Specific, Measurable, Attainable, Realistic and Time-framed. Put simply, by analysing how to reach your end goal, you increase your chances of achieving it.

**Specific** – Write down how much weight you want to lose. Is there also a particular reason you want to lose this amount, for a special occasion, or is it for health reasons? It's important to think around the reasons you want to slim down as part of the 'why' of your goal. Once it's clear in your head, you'll be in control and focused.

**Measurable** – How will you measure your weight loss? By weighing yourself regularly or by dropping a clothing size? Or will you just go by the way you look or feel? How often will you take stock of your achievements? There's no right or wrong answer here – it's just about what works for you.

**Attainable** – Question yourself as to whether this goal is really what you want. You could think about it in terms of your commitment and enthusiasm. If you're not 100% happy about your goal, maybe you need to revisit the specifics to review whether it is too ambitious or too challenging for you to feel confident about it.

**Realistic** – Think about your goal in terms of being the best you can be.

**Time-framed** – A time frame keeps your goal on track. Set a start point, such as 'I will start my healthy eating weight loss plan on Thursday' and give yourself an end time too, such as 'I will lose five kilos by my summer holiday.' I think it also makes sense to include a couple of time frames in your overall goal representing short and longer term achievements.

By now your goal should be looking so clear that you can reach out and touch it.

*Defining idea*

'*To begin with the end in mind means to start with a clear understanding of your destination.*'
**STEPHEN COVEY**

# 5. Get the write habit

**Why keeping a diary helps you lose weight**

Noting down what you are eating may give you some surprises. It will definitely help you to identify the changes you need to make to help you to lose weight.

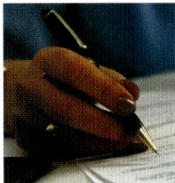

## Defining idea

*'My doctor told me to stop having intimate dinners for four. Unless there are three other people.'*
**ORSON WELLES**

All too often we're not realistic about what and how much we really eat. Sometimes we truly forget.

Sometimes we're in denial and it's simply easier to forget, to assuage feelings of guilt, self-loathing or defeatism (all common negative attitudes when you're trying to lose weight). Unless you know where you're going wrong, how can you put things right? The food diary doesn't lie – unless you cheat, of course. All you have to do is record faithfully everything you eat and drink for a week.

At the end of the week, take time to really study your diary and ask yourself the following questions:

- Am I eating regularly (breakfast, lunch and dinner)? Skipping proper meals is not a good way to lose weight.
- How often am I eating between meals and what am I grazing on? This could be because you are skipping meals, or are you snacking a lot as well as eating regular meals?
- Is my diet sufficiently varied? Does your diary tell you that you're eating the same foods day in, day out? And what types of food are they? We need a variety of foods for optimum health as well

as keeping our taste buds interested. Check the mix in your meals. Do they include a variety of different food groups on a daily basis?

■ Do I rely on junk food, takeaways and ready-prepared meals?

Our lives are busy, but if you eat this way all the time, weight gain is inevitable due to the high fat and calorie content of these types of food. You can improve on convenience and fast foods by serving your own vegetables or salads as an accompaniment.

■ What am I drinking? Alcohol, fizzy drinks and even fruit juice contain sugars that make it easy to pile on the pounds. Water is not only calorie free but also helps you to absorb nutrients from food.

Now make a list of what you could change and how you'll do it. Start with the simplest change and implement them quickly so you'll feel encouraged.

### Here's an idea for you...

Visualisation techniques are used by high achievers in many demanding fields such as sport and business. It is a proven psychological method of helping you to attain your goals. For a few minutes every day, picture yourself achieving your goals and how you'll feel and look when you've achieved them. Don't laugh – it works for Olympic gold medal winners!

# 6. Takeaway tips

**The road to Fatville is paved with fast food, but you don't have to cut it out of your life completely.**

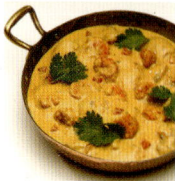

Eating takeaways and other fast foods is the norm for many of us. With little or no washing up to do, no shopping and cooking, this way of eating can feel like a life-saver for busy people. The trouble is that when you eat fast food you have no idea what you're really consuming in terms of fat, calories, hidden salt and additives, which is bad news for your health and diet.

### Fish and chips

*The good bits:* high in protein, vitamins B6 and B12, plus a few minerals.

*The bad bits:* high in fat, low on fibre. If it's a big portion, you could quite easily be consuming half the daily recommended fat levels in one sitting.

*Try this:* balance out your other meal of the day with a vitamin-packed salad and some low-fat protein, such as cottage cheese, skinless chicken or tuna.

**Pizza**

*The good bits:* cheese and tomato offers protein, calcium and some vitamins.

*The bad bits:* if you go for pepperoni and extra cheese, you're piling on fat.

*Try this:* balance out the pizza at your next meal with a chicken casserole and lots of vegetables for low-fat protein and plenty of fibre and vitamins.

**Beef burger, fries and a milkshake**

*The good bits:* high in protein, carbohydrates and calcium, plus some vitamin A, B12 and riboflavin.

*The bad bits:* high in saturated fat and sodium, low in fibre, and often a good sprinkling of additives.

*Try this:* a home-made burger is easily made with lean mince. Serve it with potato wedges and salad and either leave out the bap or use half a wholemeal roll.

When you order a takeaway to eat at home, follow the advice above plus the following tips for cutting down on calories and fat overload:

- Avoid anything fried and choose grilled, steamed, broiled or baked foods without cheese and creamy sauce.
- Say no to all creamy and buttery sauces. Choose tomato-based ones.

Here's an idea for you...

Why not choose soup as a starter? All that liquid fills you up and means there's less room for the temptation of garlic bread with cheese and bacon or 'Death by Chocolate' fudge cake.

25

- Watch out for coconut. It seems innocuous, but it's full of saturated fat.
- If you're having a side order of rice, ask for it plain boiled.

Here's a final thought: Stop eating when you're full!

# 7. Fat friends and foes

**Fats: the good, the bad and the downright ugly**

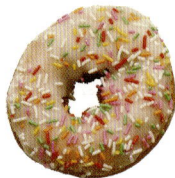

Eating too much of certain fats is definitely harmful to your waistline, so perform a bit of liposuction to your diet. Fat isn't all bad; our bodies need it. It delivers vitamins A, D, E and K and aids their absorption. It helps to regulate a variety of bodily functions. It makes food taste delicious. The thing is not all fats are created equal and we typically consume too much of the wrong kind of fat and not enough of the good stuff. So here are the big fat facts to chew on:

## Saturated fats

Foods with high levels of saturated fatty acids include butter, lard, whole milk, hard cheeses, cream, meat and meat products, palm oil and coconut oil. These are the diet wreckers and you should aim to have only a very small amount of them in your daily diet. You can reduce your intake of these kinds of fats by buying leaner cuts of meat and chopping off visible fat. Grilling, baking or steaming foods is a more slimming way to cook than smothering everything in butter and cream.

### Here's an idea for you...

Reach for the extra virgin. A drizzle a day might just keep the doctor away. The trouble is that I tend to use lots of it. Yes, it's a healthy oil, but if you eat a lot of it you are just adding unnecessary calories. The key is to measure it out. A tablespoon is usually enough.

## Trans fats

These are found in processed foods such as crisps, cakes, biscuits and pies and also in many brands of margarine. Cross the street to avoid them. Check food labels for these fats – they'll be listed as 'hydrogenated'.

## Unsaturated fats

These break down into monounsaturates and polyunsaturates. Monounsaturates are found in olive oil, nut oils, avocados and seeds, which have health benefits for your heart and so are a better choice than saturated fats. But they're still fattening, so use them sparingly.

Polyunsaturates pop up in most vegetable oils (corn, sunflower, safflower), fish oils and oily fish. They are generally a good thing, particularly if you consume them in place of saturated fats, although they are still calorific.

Average women of a healthy weight, should aim for 70 g and men 95 g. When you're trying to lose weight you should be aiming lower. For example, if you are eating around 1800 calories a day, you should go for around 63 g of fat in your diet.

# 8. Why size matters

**It's not just what you eat that counts on the road to losing weight, it's about how much you eat too.**

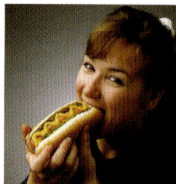

The simple fact is that most of us eat too much but portion control is essential to weight loss. You could be eating all the right things and still gain weight because you're overeating.

Here's a checklist of the sorts of foods we should be eating for a healthy balance of nutrients. It gives a range for the number of daily servings (e.g. 6–11 servings). The upper end of the range is really intended only for a very active man; most of us, especially sedentary women, should look to the lower end. It helps to get good at estimating a portion by eye because you can't carry around a set of scales everywhere you go.

Here's an idea for you...

Squeeze a lemon. Citrus fruits are a great source of vitamin C and also a phytonutrient called limonoids, which can help to lower cholesterol. These phytonutrients are concentrated in the rind, so try to incorporate the zest of citrus fruits into your cooking. They work especially well in sauces and garnishes.

**Bread, cereal, rice and pasta** – 6–11 servings
A serving is:
1 slice of bread (the size of an audio cassette tape)
1 small bread roll
2 heaped tablespoons of boiled rice
3 heaped tablespoons of boiled pasta
2 crispbreads
2 egg-sized potatoes
3 tablespoons of dry porridge oats

**Fruit and vegetables** – 2–4 servings of the former, 3–5 servings of the latter

This is based on US recommendations. In the UK, the suggested amount of fruit and vegetables is 'at least 5' a day.

A serving is:

2–3 small pieces of fruit, such as plums

1 heaped tablespoon of dried fruit such as raisins

1 medium-sized piece of fresh fruit such as half of a grapefruit or a melon

1 side salad, the size of a cereal bowl

3 heaped tablespoons of cooked vegetables such as carrots

**Meat, fish, eggs, nuts, dry beans**

2–3 servings

A serving is:

60–90 g (2–3 ounces) of cooked lean meat, poultry or fish. This is the size of a deck of cards or the palm of your hand.

150 g (5 ounces) of white fish (or three fish fingers)

120 g (4 ounces) of soya, tofu or quorn

5 tablespoons of beans

2 tablespoons of nuts and nut products

**Milk, yoghurt and cheese**
2–3 servings
A serving is:
200 ml milk
1 small pot of yoghurt
90 g (3 ounces) of cottage cheese
30 g (1 ounce) of cheddar or other
hard cheese. This is roughly the size of a matchbox.

*Defining idea*
'Never eat what you can't lift.'
**MISS PIGGY**

# 9. Body image

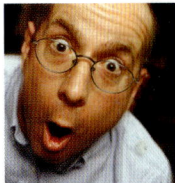

**Having a poor body image is a surefire way to sabotage your diet, so shape up with a little self-love.**

Loving yourself makes losing weight easier. This is not easy in a society that prizes slimness and makes negative judgements about people who are overweight. It's a prejudice that finds its way into the workplace and relationships, eating right into your self-esteem. The issue intensifies if hating the way you look turns into a negative view of your personality and character. 'I'm fat and stupid' or 'I'm not worth anything, no one likes me' are examples of this kind of dangerous auto-suggestion.

## Here's an idea for you...

Dieters often wear black from head to toe because it is 'slimming', but adding touches of colour can really lift your mood. Use red for energy, blue for communication, green for emotional encounters, yellow for intellectual sharpness and purple when you want to appear calm.

If you don't like yourself, it is going to be really hard to make the lifestyle changes that will help you lose weight. Often these sorts of thoughts are coupled with the habit of comparing yourself with others, especially with images in the media of celebrities and models. The truth is that these people's lives depend on how they look and they have the time and money to spend on an array of products, services and people who will keep them looking fabulous. What's more, the images you see are often 'improved' – for example, photos of models are often airbrushed to remove 'flaws'. For most of us, comparing ourselves to the thin and famous is just going to be a recipe for misery. That's rule number one: don't do it.

You need to develop a more realistic picture of how you would like to look: to look like you, but in better shape. Once you have done that, you can try some other self-esteem boosting tricks. Try writing down all the things you like about yourself, then turning them into positive statements and saying them to yourself every day like a mantra. If that seems too hard, ask your friends or family to write down what they love about you. You never know, you might finish up discovering things you had never dreamt of that will warm the cockles of your heart.

Finally, rather than seeing your body as a collection of parts that you think are awful or could use improvement, focus on it as a whole and think of the wonderful things you have done or will do with it. Cuddle someone, run a marathon, give birth, climb trees, build something, help old ladies across the road...it's your list, you finish it.

*Defining idea*

*'God made a very obvious choice when he made me voluptuous: why would I go against what he decided for me? My limbs work, so I'm not going to complain about the way my body is shaped.'*
**DREW BARRYMORE**

# 10. Can beauty products help you slim?

**Lotions, potions and treatments promise all kinds of miracles, including inch loss and wobble firming. But are they worth the money?**

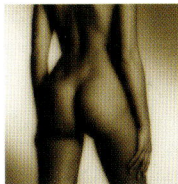

It's an appealing idea. Rub in this cream twice a day for six weeks and your flab will melt away. But to lose weight, you have to watch what you eat as well when you are spending money on some gimmicky product. The cosmetics industry is always able to produce clinical studies proving that X cream really does help you lose

Here's an idea for you...

A fake tan can make you look slimmer and leaner by sculpting, shadowing and highlighting muscles and curves. For the best results, have it applied in a salon. It will usually last for about five days.

inches, refine your silhouette or firm your curves. Meanwhile, most doctors and scientists will say that what you apply from the outside doesn't make a blind bit of difference. So it can be hard to find out how effective these products really are.

I believe that some of these treatments do have an effect, though it might be short-lived. I also think that the psychological element can't be underestimated. There's no doubt that looking after yourself does make you feel good. When you feel good, you're motivated, positive and confident, which is how you need to feel to spur you on to losing weight.

Here are our opinions of what's on offer:

**Salon treatments**
These usually involve being wrapped, massaged or painlessly zapped with some sort of electrical current. Massage is undoubtedly soothing and is claimed to stimulate your lymphatic system, which drains waste fluid from your tissues. You'll feel good afterwards, but not thinner. Wraps can shrink inches, but it's just fluid loss – they are fab for feeling a bit thinner for a special occasion. You can't beat

them for a short-term boost.
Electrical impulses stimulate your
muscles by working them while
you lie back and read a magazine.
You would see better results with
regular exercise.

*Defining idea*

'After forty a woman has to choose
between losing her figure or her face.
My advice is to keep your face and
stay sitting down.'
**BARBARA CARTLAND**

## Fat-busting creams

Despite the claims, I really don't believe you get results unless you
eat less and move more too. Still, they do make your skin feel very
smooth and soft and strokable.

## Colonic irrigation

This is very controversial. It is based on the principle that toxic
deposits are stored in your large intestine. When these are flushed
out, it kickstarts the metabolism and helps elimination. If having a
speculum inserted in your anus and having gallons of water sloshing
around your insides is your idea of a good time, go right ahead!
While many alternative practitioners say it's perfectly safe and even
emotionally rewarding, conventional doctors reject the idea, even
saying it's downright dangerous.

# 11. Snooze and lose

**What has sleep got to do with weight loss? A lot more than you probably think. So get your pyjamas on. I'll tuck you in and explain.**

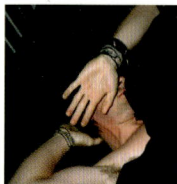

Research in the US has revealed that people who don't get enough sleep are more likely to go for high-sugar, high-fat foods and drink. The idea is that if you're not getting energy from rest, your body will encourage you to turn to quick-energy food.

*Here's an idea for you...*
Did you know a large full-fat latte packs in a hefty 260 calories? A cappuccino with skimmed milk has only 100 calories while black coffee is virtually calorie-free. Which one do you usually choose?

If you're not getting enough sleep on a prolonged basis, it could interfere with your body's ability to metabolise carbohydrates by up to 40%, according to another US study. So if you've been feeling tired, sluggish and rather peckish all day, check your 'sleep hygiene' as the sleep scientists like to call it.

**Five suggestions for better sleep**
- Keep your bedroom for sleeping. Try not to take work to bed, eat in bed or even watch TV in bed. TV encourages snacking and also doesn't create a restful atmosphere. Your bedroom should

be a comfortable temperature, dark and quiet.

■ Stimulants such as alcohol and caffeine are best avoided before bedtime. They might not wake you up, but will affect the quality of your sleep and leave you hungry for high-calorie snacks the next day.

■ Keep to a regular bedtime and waking up time whenever possible. If you're sleeping badly, it might be worth forgetting the weekend lie-ins, since they will interfere with your body's natural rhythm.

■ If your partner snores or next door's cats like to serenade you at night, try earplugs.

■ When your mind races or you feel stressed out and anxious, visualise yourself putting your worries in a drawer and locking it, telling yourself you'll deal with it in the morning.

*Defining idea...*

'Being seriously overweight – with a body mass index of 30 or more – affects breathing and increases sleep apnoea, a condition in which the airflow is cut off, breathing stops, and the brain sends panic messages to the diaphragm... As well as disrupting your sleep, it puts severe strain on your heart.'

**MICHAEL VAN STRATEN, author of The Good Sleep Guide**

*Defining idea...*

'Early to bed and early to rise makes a man healthy, wealthy and wise.'

**BENJAMIN FRANKLIN**

# 12. Suck it out

**Here's what you need to know about cosmetic surgery.**

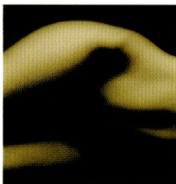

If you don't like your long toes, you can get them shortened. You can swap an 'outie' belly button for an 'innie'. You can even buy J Lo's bottom for yourself. Surgery is not a good alternative to eating less and being active, which is the safe and sensible approach to weight control. But if you have lost lots of weight and the fat loss has left you with loose rolls of skin, a tummy tuck might give you a confidence boost. The most important thing is to do lots of research, ask questions and find the best possible surgeon – you want somebody who is very experienced in your chosen op.

## Here's an idea for you...

Try an instant image change with a haircut. Layers can make your face look slimmer as can highlights. For men, a short, sharp haircut can make you look more George Clooney than Billy Bunter. Great hair works wonders.

## What surgery is on offer?

One option for fat removal is liposuction, where a narrow metal tube is inserted into the fatty area via an incision in your skin. The surgeon moves the tube back and forth and sucks out the fat with a vacuum pump, leaving the nerves and blood vessels intact. There are variations in techniques, but that's the general idea. There is a maximum amount of fat that can be removed from an area, so you might not be able to sculpt off as much as you like. It also doesn't affect cellulite (the lumpy, dimply bane of many women's lives) and can leave skin loose. Following the procedure, your skin usually

*Defining idea*

'I can spend hours in a grocery store. I get so excited when I see food, I go crazy.'
**CAMERON DIAZ**

retracts and is bruised and uncomfortable. Healing can take a long time, with lumpiness and swelling taking up to six months to disappear. It's definitely not for the faint-hearted. Neither is a tummy tuck (abdominoplasty). With this procedure, excess skin and fat can be removed and muscles tightened. There are mini, standard and extended versions. All leave a scar, from a low one at the level of the pubic hair to one that extends around to the back.

The latest high-tech techniques include LipoSelection by Vaser, which uses advanced ultrasound technology to separate out the fatty tissue from the rest before it is removed. This is claimed to be more

*Defining idea*

'I was going to have cosmetic surgery until I noticed that the doctor's office was full of portraits by Picasso.'
**RITA RUDNER**

precise, gentler and less painful, with a quicker recovery time. There is also the lower body lift, which pulls up all your slack skin around the hips, thighs and stomach. It is claimed to smooth out cellulite, flattening lumpy 'orange-peel' skin. You can also get arm and breast lifts.

# 13. Makeover your trolley

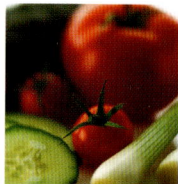

**You can save yourself pounds (££s and lbs!) by shopping wisely.**

Haphazard shopping will cost you dear in the weight-loss stakes. Here are some things to think about:

■ Do not go shopping when you're hungry. Your eyes will be seduced by all the high-fat, calorie-rich possibilities on offer, while your body says 'feed me, I'm hungry, feed me now'.

■ Take a list. That way, you'll buy everything you really need and minimise the threat of impulse buys.

■ Check the labels to see what you're really getting. Low fat only counts if it is 3 g or less per 100 g. Avoid special offers, super-sizes and multi-buys unless they're healthy and low fat.

A trip around the aisles should end up looking something like this:

**Things to put in the trolley**

■ Wholegrains – they're not less calorific than white, refined produce, but they have more fibre and will keep you feeling full for longer

■ Lots of colourful fruit and vegetables

- Low-fat dairy produce
- Lean cuts of meat, chicken and turkey (the white meat is lower in fat than dark)
- Fish, including a portion or two of oily fish, such as salmon, tuna, mackerel and herring
- Dried fruit to snack on – it's calorific, but OK if you keep servings small; low-fat/reduced-calorie cereal
- Low fat and cereal snack bars – but still check the label for the better buys

### Here's an idea for you...

Chop bananas into bite-sized chunks and freeze them. They then become healthy, delicious, almost ice-creamy treats to snack on. You can freeze grapes too or make your own ice lollies by freezing fruit juice.

### Things to leave on the shelf

- Cereals with added sugar (pick out the sugar-free ones and choose oats if you like porridge or making your own muesli)
- Biscuits and cakes, crisps
- Sausages, meat pies and pasties
- Anything with pastry
- Battered and bread-crumbed meat and seafood (all that extra fat and calories)
- Jams and spreads (choose sugar-free versions)
- Full fat ice-cream – why not try frozen yoghurt instead?

# 14. It's my allergy

**Food allergies and intolerances are very real. They can be fatal. But can they make you fat or is it just a fashionable excuse?**

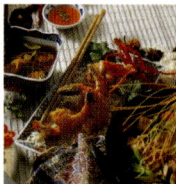

Lots of people latch on to the latest fad in allergies to justify their poor eating habits, which does not do them, or the genuine sufferers, any favours. Years ago I had a raft of food allergy tests because it was the late 80s and it was 'in' to blame weight gain on certain foods. Apparently if I gave up courgettes I would lose that extra half stone I wanted to shift. Give them up? We were barely on first name terms! It was a waste of time and money.

A proper food allergy occurs when your body responds to a substance with an immunological reaction. That is, it releases histamine and other chemicals into your bloodstream to fight the invader.

### Defining idea

*'I'm allergic to food. Every time I eat it, I break out in fat.'*
**JENNIFER GREENE DUNCAN**

Food intolerances don't involve an immunological reaction, but can still be unpleasant. They include enzyme defects. For example, a lactose deficiency makes you unable to digest lactose, the milk sugar, and can cause various bowel problems and migraines. You can also suffer pharmacological reactions in response to various components of food, such as amines in coffee and chocolate. Your symptoms can be anything from migraines to anxiety, to aching muscles or water retention. You know there's something wrong, but nine times out of ten your doctor will say you just have to live with it.

## Here's an idea for you...

In a study on laughter, one group sat quietly in a room while another group watched a stand-up comic. Blood samples taken later showed that the group who had been laughing had reduced cortisol, the stress hormone linked to weight gain.

With all of these, it's essential to be properly diagnosed by a doctor or nutritionist who can do various sensitivity tests and help you with a food elimination diet where you cut out what you think you could be sensitive to and gradually reintroduce it, watching for a reaction.

All of these issues are very real, but various diet gurus and alternative health practitioners jump on the food intolerance bandwagon and say if you only give up X and Y, you'll not only feel fantastic, but drop loads of excess weight into the bargain. Not true! It is hard to lose weight. It takes time, discipline and lifestyle changes. The desire to lose weight also makes you vulnerable to quackery; how reassuring it is to be told that your

## Defining idea

'Given that the most common sources of food intolerance are wheat and milk, such therapists can achieve a reasonable success rate by diagnosing sensitivity to these two foods in all their patients.'
**JONATHAN BROSTOFF, *The Complete Guide to Food Allergy and Intolerance***

weight problem has nothing to do with anything except your intolerance to, say, wheat or dairy products.

Concentrate on tried and tested methods of weight loss.

# 15. Diet doctor

**The Atkins diet and its imitators are as controversial as they are popular. Does it work and is it safe?**

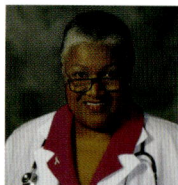

### The Atkins theory

If you eat a lot of carbohydrates, insulin is released which encourages the body to store the energy from food as fat. Eventually you can be 'insulin resistant', which means your body releases very high levels of insulin just to maintain normal blood sugar levels, encouraging more fat to be stored. Switching to low levels of carbohydrate intake leads your body to burn fat as its energy source, rather than glucose from carbohydrates. Eating fat doesn't affect your blood sugar and, contrary to popular opinion, can be good for your health. Fat also helps you to feel satisfied after eating.

## In practice

The Atkins diet requires you to start on an induction plan that lasts a minimum of fourteen days. It's pretty strict, including rules such as eating no more than 20 g of carbohydrates a day, which should come from salad greens and certain other 'acceptable' vegetables; no fruit, bread, grains or dairy foods other than cheese, cream and butter; plenty of poultry, fish and meat; no caffeine, processed foods and refined sugars. As you progress, you move through another three phases, culminating in your lifetime maintenance plan. Each phase changes what you can and can't eat; for instance, later on you eat less fat than in the beginning.

You have to follow the diet to the letter or it won't work, and it's not for the short term – it's a way of eating for life.

## What's the verdict?

It works for some people. Critics have raised concerns about high fat intakes because of the risk of heart disease, but there are studies that show that the diet can have a

### Defining idea

'The perfect diet for those who love food.'
**NIGELLA LAWSON**

### Defining idea

'Atkins has never been about no carbs. It's about choosing the right carbs in the right amount.'
**Dr STUART TRAGER, Medical Director of Atkins Nutritionals Inc.**

Here's an idea for you...

Try a carb curfew. Pioneered by British health and fitness expert Joanna Hall, the rule is to eat no carbs after five o'clock. It's a neat way to avoid excess carbohydrates, cuts some calories, and you don't go to bed feeling bloated.

beneficial effect on cholesterol levels and fats in the blood in the longer term. Kidney damage is another charge levelled at the diet, but there's no real proof. Atkins makes it clear that the diet is not for those who have kidney disease, or for pregnant women and nursing mothers. If you're diabetic, speak to your doctor about the diet. Diabetics can follow the Atkins diet, but only under very careful medical supervision.

# 16. Time for tea

**It's a seductive idea: sip tea and watch the weight melt away. But can tea ever really be more than a refreshing drink?**

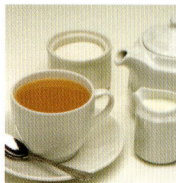

Let me read your tea-leaves. I see a large shape saying this cup of diet tea was a waste of time. Stick to sensible eating and more exercise instead of lying around drinking your brew of 'Bye Bye Fat'. We all like an easy option, and what could be easier than sipping yourself slim with a fat-busting tea? Health food stores offer some of these super-charged brews, but it's on the internet that you're really spoiled for choice. And it's also on the internet that you can say or sell just about anything you want and get away with it. As with many things in life, not everything is what it seems, and tea is no exception.

Green tea has been in the spotlight recently, following various research projects. It has been linked with having a preventative effect on all kinds of diseases, including certain cancers, as well as having the ability to lower cholesterol and to speed up fat oxidation, i.e. to burn calories quicker. Further research is needed but it's safe to say that if you like the taste of green tea, you've got nothing to lose apart from just possibly a few kilos and much to gain in health benefits.

**Tried and trusted?**

Diet teas, which contain ingredients such as licorice root, senna and buckthorn, should really be called laxative teas because

Defining idea

*'Drinking a daily cup of tea will surely starve the apothecary.'*
**CHINESE PROVERB**

that's what they do to you! Others act as diuretics, especially if they have dandelion, parsley or juniper as ingredients, so you lose water weight. Then there are the diet teas that contain stimulants such as yerba mate, kola nut and guarana. They're OK in small doses, but if you're sensitive to the ingredients or have just a little too much, you'll get palpitations, the jitters and have difficulty sleeping. It's rare, but there's a risk of heart attack. Since the only reason you'll be drinking the teas that are marketed as slimming aids is to lose weight (most of them don't actually taste that great) and as there's absolutely no proof that they can help, I'd leave them well alone. Stick to a nice cup of real tea, or traditional herbal tea that doesn't make any other claim than it tastes good!

# 17. Couldn't I just pop a pill?

**You would think there would be a safe, effective, fat-reducing pill that you could buy at the pharmacy. Some would say it's already here in the form of supplements and prescription drugs. So what's the truth?**

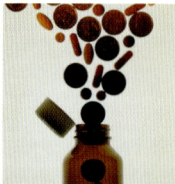

There are many supplements that promise appetite suppression, weight loss and increases in lean muscle mass. These products are widely available through pharmacies, health food stores and of course the good old internet. Often you might find a trainer at your local gym recommending them too. But do any of them actually

work? Let's look at a few of the
most popular:

**Here's an idea for you...**

It's early days, but scientists have
isolated the active molecules in the
*Hoodia gordonii* plant, used by
tribesmen in the Kalahari to stave off
hunger pangs while on hunting trips.
Some products are already available,
being sold as appetite suppressants and
anecdotally are getting good reviews.
However, more research is needed.

**Chromium picolinate** The lure of
supplements that combine
chromium and picolinate is the
potential of losing fat and gaining
muscle tone – this is based on the
results of a number of studies.
However, further research hasn't
been able to duplicate the original
claims and indeed some research has subsequently made links
between high levels of supplementation, DNA damage and a host of
other nasties. In fact, at the time of writing, this substance is facing
a ban in the UK.

**Chitosan** This is made from crushed crab and lobster shells! The
theory is that the fibre from the shells binds with the fat from your
food before it is metabolised. Chitosan will decrease the absorption
of fat-soluble vitamins, plus you'll experience a laxative effect. It is
not recommended – especially if you're allergic to shellfish!

**Amino acids** These are readily available as pills and powders, but
despite the hype there's no proof that they will increase muscle
mass or burn fat as a supplement. You are better off with protein
foods such as meat and eggs and plenty of exercise.

## Defining idea

'People usually spend more time researching their next car or computer purchase than selecting their supplements.'
**FELICIA BUSCH, *The New Nutrition***

### Doctor's orders

Producing a weight-control pill is truly one of the Holy Grails of pharmaceutical companies, because anything that even half works is a veritable goldmine. There are already products available. You may have heard of sibutramine, marketed as Reductil, and Orlistat (or Xenical) to name a couple. Trials of a drug called Rimonabant have also been successful in both weight loss and helping smokers to quit without piling on pounds. At the moment the drugs that are licensed can only be given to you on prescription from your doctor.

In conclusion, beware of supplements that promise weight loss and muscle tone with no effort. At best they just won't work and will be a waste of money. At worst, they could be dangerous.

# 18. Spot reduction

**How much can you change your natural shape? Is it possible to lose weight from specific areas of your body? There are many myths surrounding those questions. Here's the truth.**

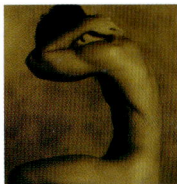

We either have an android or gynoid influence. The android is an apple shape, with most weight carried on the top half of the body (and of course, sooner or later around the abdominal area). The gynoid influence, which is a pear shape, i.e. heavier on the bottom half, is a more female shape. The key is to identify the closest to your shape and work with it, rather than battling against it, to be in the best possible shape you can be.

*Here's an idea for you...*

To get an idea of whether you really need to lose weight or indeed to track your progress, you can have your body fat measured electronically. A harmless electric current is passed through your body which estimates body water, showing the amount of muscle you have. The difference between your overall weight and lean tissue weight gives an idea of your body fat. Gyms and health centres usually offer this service (for a price) or you can also buy special scales to use at home.

**Movers and shapers**

You cannot spot reduce and lose weight from specific areas of the body. Research has shown that we all tend to lose weight from the

## Defining idea

*'I'm in shape. Round is a shape, isn't it?'*
**ANONYMOUS**

top down, so, first it shows in your face, then your chest and stomach area, followed by hips, thighs and legs. Abdominal fat seems to be fairly easy to shift – good news for apple shapes, less good for pear shapes. But of course as abdominal fat is a risk factor in heart disease, pear shaped people can afford to be a little smug. But I'd rather be slim and in proportion, I hear the pear shapes say. A fat pear shaped person will slim into, well, a slimmer pear shaped person. And there's not a lot more you can do about your basic shape apart from surgery, which I don't recommend. There is also exercise, which I do strongly recommend. One of the best tips for the pear-shaped person is to focus your strength training efforts on your top half to create more balance.

How much can exercise change your shape? Toning exercises certainly work to either increase your muscle bulk or streamline your muscles. However, if you've got lots of fat covering your muscles it will be harder to see muscle definition, plus you could just end up looking bigger. It's best to lose some body fat first. Contrary to popular myth it's not possible to turn fat into muscle or the other way around. Fat is fat and muscle is muscle.

# 19. Confidence tricks

**You don't have to be beautiful to be perceived as such. Start with a few self-esteem tricks.**

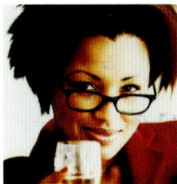

Many of those who aren't skinny exude a goddess-like aura nevertheless. This is more than 'charm' and less obvious than raw sex appeal, although they may have that too. It's an intrinsic self-belief and joie de vivre that makes even 'homely' women somehow magnetic. Some people have bags of it. It may be something they were lucky enough to acquire in childhood. However, if you didn't acquire it, you don't need hours of therapy to get some too. Self-confidence (real or faked) is a beauty trick we can all learn.

Life coaches and shrinks suggest we tell ourselves at every opportunity how fantastic we are. Most of us cringe at the thought, however, so I suggest listing your hottest qualities instead. Go on. Get a piece of paper and list them under a heading such as 'Things I Like About Myself' or 'My Best Bits'. An alternative is to make a list of all the compliments you've received. In moments of self-doubt, consult your list.

Second, start focusing on and pampering the bits you love about yourself. So, if you've been told you have great legs, then capitalise

## Here's an idea for you...

Fill a photo album with pictures of yourself looking your best and reach for it whenever low self-confidence is a problem.

on that. For example, indulge in some amazingly expensive body oil for them, buy yourself some unspeakably impractical but undeniably fuck-me shoes or add a few new leg-revealing mini skirts or floaty numbers to your wardrobe.

Pampering yourself on a regular basis is a great way to boost your self-confidence. How much more attractive do you feel after a facial/manicure or even after a spritz of a new perfume? Start taking pleasure in looking your best.

## Defining idea

*'Life's not about finding yourself. Life is about creating yourself.'*
**GEORGE BERNARD SHAW**

But what if you're overweight/out of shape/flabbier than you were two, five or ten years ago? Well, you have two options here. First, do all the above. Second, throw out your thin clothes (they'll only depress you) and get a completely new wardrobe of clothes that fit and flatter you.

I'd suggest that you start doing some exercise as well. Simply moving your body regularly can help boost your mood, improve your complexion and give you confidence in your shape. And before you know it you'll have lost pounds! Aim for about twenty minutes of exercise three times a week. If you start to see it as a chore remind yourself that you're doing something positive to make the best of your shape and see it as a short cut to self-belief instead.

# 20. Water works

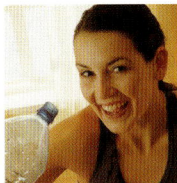

**Water is a beauty tonic on tap. Eight glasses a day can boost your energy and make you slimmer, cleverer and more positive.**

Water is involved in nearly every bodily function, from circulation to body temperature and from digestion to waste excretion. It helps your body to absorb the nutrients from food, too. When you get dehydrated, vitamins and minerals aren't absorbed optimally and toxins can't get excreted as efficiently. And, when you're not getting enough water, your blood volume drops, which stops you from firing on all cylinders.

So, how much water do we really need? The Natural Mineral Water Information Service estimates that about 90% of us don't get enough fluids. Your best gauge is the colour of your urine. You're after a pale watery colour with a tinge of lemon; yellow urine means you need to drink more.

## Here's an idea for you...

Eat up your fluids, too. Fruit and vegetables are largely water – apricots, grapes, melons, peaches, strawberries, cucumbers, mangoes, oranges and peppers all comprise over 75% water. Fish such as sardines, mackerel, salmon and tuna is also 50% water.

If you're partying, match a glass of water for every alcoholic drink. And drink at least half a cup of water for each drink containing caffeine (such as tea, coffee or cola) to counteract the diuretic effect. Sipping is better than gulping huge glasses at a time. Experts say that the latter is just like pouring water on a dry leaf, so certainly not the best way to absorb it.

## Water can help you lose weight

How often do you confuse hunger with thirst and end up reaching for food instead of drinking? This is very common, but will cost you dearly in calories. Research shows that 75% of all hunger pangs are actually thirst pangs, so if you get the munchies and fancy a Mars Bar, try a glass of water instead and save yourself some calories. One study showed that you could increase your metabolic rate by about 30% by having a big 500 ml glass of cold water after each meal. This comes down to a process called thermogenesis, in other words the rate at which your body burns calories for digestion. Apparently, drinking cold water means you'll

## Defining idea

'Beauty of style and harmony and grace and good rhythm depend on simplicity.'
**PLATO**

burn off your supper that much quicker! In fact, one study found that drinking 2 litres of water daily can help your body to burn off an extra 150 calories a day. This can also flatten your tum because it can help you beat the water retention that causes bloated bellies.

# 21. Lose pounds without trying

**A few simple lifestyle changes may be all you need to drop a dress size.**

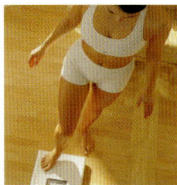

The year I gave up dieting I lost more weight than I'd ever managed before.

Diets don't work because they're offering short-term solutions that are impossible to sustain in the long term. You either feel so hungry, deprived or bored that you instantly crave that which you're not allowed or your nutrition is so unbalanced that your body steers you towards the calories it craves.

*Here's an idea for you...*

Beware buffets: experts say that if you're presented with a large variety of foods you tend to eat more.

So, here are five golden rules of healthy eating that really will help you to shed pounds without suffering:

## Defining idea

*'I feel about airplanes the way I feel about diets. It seems to me that they are wonderful things for other people to go on.'*
**JEAN KERR, Writer**

### 1. Don't skip breakfast

Skipping breakfast won't help you to save calories and lose pounds. On the contrary, when you do eat breakfast you're more likely to make better, lower-calorie choices throughout the rest of the day because it'll kick-start your metabolism.

### 2. Eat lots of fibre

One study showed that people who ate a low-fat diet that included 26 g of fibre per 1,000 calories lost more weight than those whose diet was higher in fat and lower in fibre (just 7 g per day). Eat bran cereals, wholemeal pasta, wholemeal bread and lots of fruit and vegetables.

### 3. Be supermarket savvy

Never shop hungry and always make a list so that you're less likely to succumb to those tasty but high-fat 'two for one' offers or the crisps and chocolate at the checkout. And unless you're doing a big weekly shop, always use a basket rather than a trolley so that by the time you've bought your essentials, you can't carry anything else!

### 4.  Use smaller plates

Swap those whopping dinner plates for smaller ones about 20 cm in
diameter (a dinner plate is usually about 25–30 cm in diameter), as
people tend to clear their plates regardless of how many calories this
means they eat.

### 5.  Eat fruit or salad before meals

One study showed that women who ate a little apple or pear before
each meal lost more weight than women who skipped the fruit. In
another study, people who ate a low-fat 100-calorie salad before their
meal ate about 12% less than those who didn't have the salad.

# 22. Look great in photos

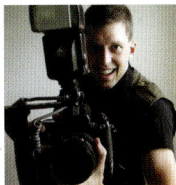

**The camera *will* lie when you want it to
help you lose weight instantly**

Sticking your tongue into the roof of your mouth will make your
lower facial muscles contract and tighten a double-chin.
Camera-shy or woefully unphotogenic people should commit this

## Here's an idea for you...

Maximise your lips. To pout beautifully, turn to the camera and say 'Wogan'. Bizarre, I know, but glamour models swear by it.

kind of tip to memory. And knowing how to show off your most beautiful features will also equip you for those horrifying times when someone feels compelled to 'capture the moment'.

- To look your slimmest try standing with one foot slightly in front of the other and gently pivot on your feet so that your body, including your shoulders, are at a slight angle. And putting your hands on your hips can make your waist look smaller.
- If you're sitting down, lean forward and rest your elbows on your knees. That way you'll disguise wobbly thighs and look slimmer.
- Brighten up. Dark colours can be slimming to wear, but black can drain the colour from the face so choose brighter colours for your top half to bring out the best in your skin tone.
- Dark circles or bags under your eyes? Try lifting your chin to avoid shadows falling on your face.
- Smile. A lovely smile really does take the focus away from the bits you're less happy with.
- Poker straight hair can pull your face down. Putting your hair up can soften your features and draw attention to your smile.
- Get the photographer to take more than one photo! The more you have taken, the more likely it is you'll be captured from a flattering angle. Remember there's safety in numbers.

**Make-up tricks**

- Apply a light foundation only where necessary, such as to the sides of your nose or over spots.
- To avoid a shiny face, stick to matte-formula make-up for your blemishes and only use creamy, reflective concealers for your eyes.
- Flatter your best features. Apply blush over the apple part of your cheeks. Never overplay the eyes and the lips. Choose between them before you open that make-up bag.

*Defining idea*

*'With charm you've got to get up close to see it; style slaps you in the face.'*

**JOHN COOPER CLARKE, poet and comedian**

# 23. Move that body

**Exercise has the potential to transform your body. And it's free!**

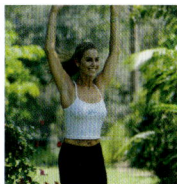

There's nothing to beat the smug knowledge that you've done something to burn calories and tone your wobbly bits.

Extraordinary things happen at a physiological level when you exercise. When you start moving, your body's endorphins – natural

## Here's an idea for you...

Couch potatoes can turn an evening vegging in front of the TV into a workout by fidgeting more, which can apparently burn up to 800 calories a day. So make a point of shifting around every fifteen minutes – adjust your posture, roll your shoulders or change the way you cross your legs. The same goes for sitting at your desk or driving,

opiates – are released, which block your body's pain receptors so you feel euphoric.

When you exercise, a growth hormone is secreted into your body, which helps thicken and firm up the skin and puts wrinkles on hold. Studies have shown that athletes' skin is thicker and contains more collagen than other people's. Experts say we should aim for a minimum of three twenty- to thirty-minute aerobic sessions per week, such as running, swimming, cycling, dancing or brisk walking. If possible, also try to add in three half-hour sessions of weight or resistance work, which increases muscle mass and can boost our body's metabolism.

If you're new to exercise, don't rush it. Start small and be realistic about what you want to achieve. Instead, focus on an event, such as having to fit into a dress. Every week aim to do something, even if it's a twenty-minute stroll every other day. Make a list of what you're going to do each week and stick to it. And try to change your approach to exercise and think of it as a way to de-stress, energise and make your skin glow and not merely 'burning calories'.

Exercise will also make you more interesting! Studies have shown that long-distance exercise such as rowing, walking, running or swimming is good for creativity because while you're doing it your brain is 'set free'. Anything over ten minutes counts.

*Defining idea*

'A bear, however hard he tries, grows tubby without exercise.'
**WINNIE THE POOH**

If you're not a natural exerciser, the key is to think in terms of activities rather than workouts as activities will sound less like a chore. Swimming, hiking, cycling, walking or rollerblading are far more appealing than going to the gym.

The key to whipping your body into shape is to make sure you build up to a variety of different forms of exercise each week. That way you're less likely to get bored, plus you'll tone up different parts of your body. So try swimming (burns almost 200 calories in half an hour), then power-walking (300 calories in half an hour), plus have an exercise-video session or do a few sets of press-ups – great for a toned bust.

# 24. Lose 10 lbs without dieting

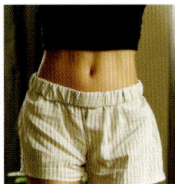

**Dress cleverly – in shades, cuts and styles to suit you. It's the simplest way to slimmer and more shapely you.**

I rarely used to dress in anything other than black, mistakenly believing that black made me look barely-there thin.

Don't get me wrong. Black can undoubtedly look supremely elegant. In fact, the longer the streak you create, the better. Black is rarely individual, however. Dark colours certainly can minimise the bulges, but it's not the only sartorial route to a more slender you. Besides, black can also be dreary and draining. And if you get it ever so slightly wrong at functions, you'll have half a dozen coats flung at you or be asked for another vol-au-vent.

## Here's an idea for you...

Colour experts say white, silver and mother of pearl are 'eternally feminine' because they're associated with the moon, stars and sea. Light colours close to your face can reflect light and take years off you.

- You can still create the illusion of being longer and leaner if you're dressed head to foot in the same shade, even white.

- Ignore size tags when you're shopping. You can lose pounds by wearing slightly looser clothes that skim over bumps.

- Where possible, choose lined clothes. They won't hug you so unforgivingly. Lined trousers are a godsend, particularly in summer, as they drop crisply, however hot and sweaty you are beneath.

- Invest in an A-line skirt. These flatter almost everyone because they don't cling to your curves but they do minimise your bottom. The best length is on or just below the knee and if you team it with knee-length boots you can disguise thick legs and hefty unfeminine thighs.

- Always wear a heel, however slight. The extra inch or two will add length and make you more aware of your posture.

- Disguise a big bust with V-necks and low scoop necks. Avoid slash necks and halter necks altogether.

- Always choose trousers with hems long enough to skim the tip of a boot or shoe. They may feel too long, but they'll immediately draw the eye down, giving the impression of a longer, leaner leg.

- Investing in good lingerie can knock pounds off you. So, go for well-fitting bras with uplift and knickers that flatten in the right places. With bras, aim to banish seams, puckering and surplus flesh bursting out of cups.

*Defining idea*

*'I have always said that the best clothes are invisible...they make you notice the person.'*
**KATHARINE HAMNETT**

# 25. Why walking works wonders

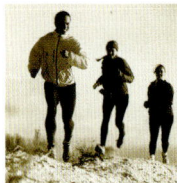

**If vigorous exercise doesn't appeal, walking might. It's a gentler alternative that'll tone bums, tums and thighs in no time.**

*Here's an idea for you...*

For best results, check your posture. Aim to keep your shoulders back and your ribcage lifted. Pull your abdominal muscles in and think tall. Look forward not down. Strike forward with your heel and push off with your back foot. You can gradually increase the length of your stride but don't overstretch.

Experts now say that if we clock up 10,000 steps a day we'll be doing all the exercise we need to keep fit. Most of us walk an average of between 2,000 and 6,000 steps a day, that's about one and three miles respectively and we do this just by walking around the office at work, going from the car to the house, strolling up and down the supermarket aisles, that kind of thing. So, walking an extra few thousand steps (about an extra half an hour a day) by upping the amount of 'incidental' walking you do can transform your health and shed pounds.

Simple isn't it? Plus all you need in terms of equipment is a pair of supportive shoes and some loose clothing. A pedometer may be an investment too, particularly if you're losing count of all those steps!

It's a little instrument that clips onto your belt and measures the number of steps you take; it costs about the same as a DVD.

**Defining idea**

*'Walking is man's best medicine.'*
**HIPPOCRATES**

Let's have a look at why walking is so great:

- It can burn up to 200 calories in half an hour. Walk up stairs for five minutes and you can burn up to 150 calories.
- Walking just 1 mile per day can significantly increase your bone density.
- Walking, even for just a few hours a week, significantly reduces your risk of breast cancer, stroke and heart disease.
- Being outside, particularly among greenery, can be great for your well-being and boosts your mood. Twenty minutes' walking will give you plenty of productive thinking time, lets you appreciate your surroundings and smell the air, and helps you put things into focus.

Consider getting off the train earlier and walking the rest of the way to work. Or parking in the furthest space from the entrance of the supermarket. Walk around while you're on the phone, bin the remote and get up to change the channel instead (this one won't work if you live with a man, of course).

# 26. Get more energy without more sleep

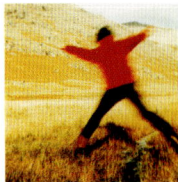

**Energy is essential for weight loss motivation**

When you're bursting with energy, your skin will look radiant, your eyes will shine and you'll generally look perky. Lose sleep, however, and you'll suffer.

### Give yourself an energy blast

Essential oils of rosemary, clary sage, orange and lemon are energising and uplifting. For a morning boost, either add a couple of drops to your bath or burn oils in a diffuser while you're showering and dressing.

## Here's an idea for you...

Brighten up your world. Colour experts say orange can be a great pick-me-up so a bowl of oranges on your desk or a vase of marigolds on the sitting-room table will perk you up in no time.

### Enjoy that morning cuppa

A cup of tea really can boost clear-headedness. Don't go overboard, however, as more than one cup of tea or coffee hasn't been found to have additional benefits in this respect.

## Eat a power breakfast

You need both protein and carbohydrates to stop your blood sugar levels from plummeting. Try eggs on toast with orange juice or a milk-based fruit smoothie with added wheatgerm.

## Supersnack

Ditch the crisps and chocolate and instead munch on flapjacks, wholemeal toast with peanut butter, mixed fruit salad with yoghurt, a bowl of high-fibre cereal with banana and nuts, humous on crackers, peanuts, apples or cherries to keep you feeling fuller and energised for longer.

## Sip water throughout the day

Water feeds every cell in your body and keeps it well fuelled. The Chinese believe that sipping gradually rather than gulping down glasses at a time is the key to constant, energising hydration.

## Have an al fresco lunch

A lack of natural light along with exposure to fluorescent light (used in most offices) can trigger your body's production of melatonin, which can make you feel mentally and physically fatigued, so get outside.

**Try herbs**

Siberian ginseng is said to help the body cope during times of stress. Experts say it can boost stamina and strength, improve brainpower and concentration, even promote longevity and strengthen immunity. Taking a supplement could help speed reaction and improve alertness and concentration within hours.

# 27. Beat the bloat

**Bloating is the bane of many women's lives. It can add pounds overnight and force you to resort to your 'fat' wardrobe.**

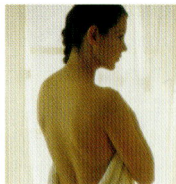

When your stomach is firm and flat the world seems a kinder, brighter place. Bloating is caused by trapped wind in your digestive system. The chief culprits range from food intolerances, constipation, too much alcohol, too much salt, eating too quickly or munching on too many gas-causing foods such as baked beans.

- Cut down on top bloaters such as wheat and replace them with rice or oats, which are usually better tolerated.
- Avoid constipation by eating plenty of fresh fruit and vegetables and drinking plenty of fluids.
- Try a course of probiotics (such as acidophilus), which can help

rebalance the good and bad bacteria in your digestive system. If the balance gets out of kilter your system will slow down, which can cause lots of gas in your gut.

*Here's an idea for you...*

Stress can cause havoc with your digestive system so aim to set aside plenty of time for quality rest and relaxation and develop some great strategies for nipping stress in the bud.

- Fill your fruit bowl. Apples, pears and rhubarb are a great source of potassium, which helps rebalance your body's fluid levels. They're also a good source of pectin, a soluble fibre that keeps you regular. Pineapples are great for beating bloat, too, as they contain the wonder-enzyme bromelain that helps digestion.
- Cut down on alcohol and salty foods, which can cause fluid retention and inflate that bloated tummy further. That's because your body holds on to fluid to dilute the extra salt. Avoid ready meals and processed foods, which often contain tons of salt.
- Eat plenty of natural diuretics to help beat water retention, including celery, onion and parsley.
- Address those PMS symptoms and if you're plagued with bloating each month, try a supplement. There's evidence that taking 1,000 mg of calcium a day (the recommended daily allowance is 700 mg) may improve problems concerning water retention.
- Drink at least eight glasses of water a day. Regular, small amounts are best.
- Slow down at mealtimes, stop eating on the run and aim to

savour your food and chew
everything thoroughly. When you
gulp your meals down you can
swallow air, which can bloat you.

■  Try some tummy-toning moves.
Pilates is a great way to work
your stomach muscles.

# 28. Get bikini fit

**Looking beautiful when wearing very little
requires specialist tactics**

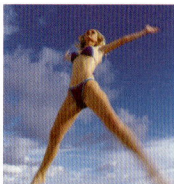

Also, there are bikini rules that can't be
broken unless you're under sixteen, Ursula Andress or model-slim
with buttocks you could crack nuts with. First, take a long look at
your body in a full-length mirror. Assess your proportions and
establish your body shape.

Now take a look at the tips below. Think of them as your cut-out-
and-keep guide to bikini shopping. The truth is, you can still wear a
bikini if you have a less than model-like body. You just need some
poolside savvy such as what cuts, colours and shapes to choose.

**Flat- or small-chested?**

The best techniques for boosting small busts include wearing padded bras and tops with frilly details or horizontal stripes. You could also try underwired bras with bows or flowers that'll add an extra dimension to an otherwise uneventful bustline.

**Pear-shaped or big-bottomed?**

Try tie-sided briefs, even if you thought you'd left them behind with your teens. They're not actually age-dependent and are flattering on bigger hips. Also, you can adjust them to fit perfectly and the ties detract from any lumps and bumps. Alternatively, choose bikinis with boyish shorts or flippy skirts.

**What about colour?**

If you're trying to minimise a curvaceous bum and enhance a smaller bust, try a solid dark colour on the bottom and put the colour and pattern on top.

### Here's an idea for you...

Before splashing out on that gorgeous new bikini, make sure it fits comfortably and is also practical. Check that it does actually contain you and your curves when you're moving by running on the spot and raising your arms up and down. Also ensure the bottoms won't ride up uncomfortably by doing a few squats or kneeling down.

### Defining idea

'There is no excellent beauty that hath not some strangeness in the proportion.'
**SIR FRANCIS BACON**

**Busty?**

There's nothing sexy about huge knockers if you own a pair of them and are trying to squeeze them into swimwear. So, in order to draw attention away from your boobs to your face and at the same time lengthen your torso, go for V-neck swimsuits or bikinis. These will draw the eye from your décolletage downwards, effectively carving your bust in two. Another good tip to minimise a hefty bust is to choose thick shoulder straps.

**Big tummy?**

Opt for vest tops with built-in support, which are great at covering a bulging tummy. Alternatively, go for high-cut bikini bottoms that come higher over your tummy.

# 29. Cellulite busting

**The moves, the creams, the treatments, the foods, the pants – one way or another, you will beat cellulite**

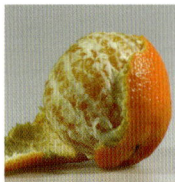

Cellulite is a reminder that life can be cruel. It afflicts nearly 85% of us – including supermodels. (Okay, so it's not always that cruel.) Fortunately there are steps you can take.

## Exercise more

Research has shown that women
who followed a low-fat diet and did
twenty minutes of aerobic exercise
weekly, including some strength
exercises, lost 3.5 kg in weight
(nearly 5 cm from their thighs).

*Here's an idea for you...*

A DIY massage is a good night-time
treatment. Gently but firmly massage
your legs and thighs using upward
movements and also a gentle kneading
motion, always working towards your
heart.

Plus 70% of women said that their cellulite improved in just six
weeks by doing weight training aimed at their legs.

When you exercise you boost your circulation and lymph drainage,
so you build muscle that effectively boosts the skin, which helps
flatten out those bumpy bits. Plus, taking more exercise – at least
twenty to thirty minutes three to five times a week – can help shift
some of the fat that causes cellulite.

Aim to do three sessions a week of aerobic exercise such as cycling,
running, dancing, kickboxing or a fitness video. Also, make sure
you're doing some resistance or strength work as building lean
muscle is vital; good moves are lunges, squats or 'step' work (cycle
uphill, try a step class or run on a treadmill at an incline).

## Watch your diet

Losing a few pounds can help reduce the fat that causes your
cellulite. Try to cut back on salt, which causes water retention, and
on fatty and sugary foods. Eat tons of fruit and vegetables, as these

## Defining idea

'The chief excitement in a woman's life is spotting women who are fatter than she is.'
**HELEN ROWLAND, writer**

are rich in antioxidants that help mop up the free radicals that can damage skin and cause wrinkles and sagging.

Aim to drink about 2 litres of water a day to help boost circulation and reduce water retention. And watch your alcohol and coffee intake, as both can interfere with your circulation.

### Body brush and pamper

Endermologie is arguably the only salon treatment that has any proven results. You'll need about ten sessions and a healthy bank account to see the results for yourself, but it could be worth a try. It's a deep-tissue massage treatment using a machine that rolls back and forth across your cellulite to break down fat cells and firm your skin. It is approved in the US by the FDA as an effective, albeit temporary, treatment for cellulite.

A cheaper option is to body brush every day. Body brushing is thought to help boost the skin's circulation and lymph flow, which can help beat the fluid build that swells your fat cells.

Start at your feet and with a brush made from natural fibres brush in long strokes (always in the direction of your heart). Ideally do it morning and night before a shower or bath.

# 30. Boost your bust

**Sadly, half of women hate their breasts, yet practically all (straight) men love them**

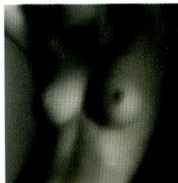

If yours are too big because you're too heavy, that doesn't help. The bottom line is, nothing short of surgery will change the shape of breasts. However, good posture and strength-building exercises can help improve the back and chest muscles and perk the whole area up considerably. Try these:

**Boob raisers**

**Press-ups** Press-ups are considered the best move for a firmer chest. Get down on your hands and knees and put your hands a little more than hip distance apart, keeping your hands in line with your shoulders. Keeping the part of your thigh just above your knees on the ground, lower your chest so that your elbows come out slightly to the side and then slowly push up again without locking them. Keep your stomach pulled in tight and don't allow your back to sag. The wider apart your hands are the more you work your chest.

Aim for three sets of ten to fifteen press-ups three times a week. Try full press-ups once you've mastered these modified ones.

## Here's an idea for you...

Get to know your breasts and take a moment in the shower to check up and down your breast and armpit area. Check for lumps or hard areas by either moving your fingers up and down or by gently pressing in a circular motion.

**The back extension** The back extension can help support your breasts and improve your posture.

After each set of push-ups, lie face down on the floor, lift one arm and the opposing leg a few inches straight in the air simultaneously and hold for a count of ten. Do this move twice on each side. Back extensions will strengthen your upper and lower back muscles, thus improving posture.

## Defining idea

'A woman without breasts is like a bed without pillows.'
**ANATOLE FRANCE, writer**

**Bust beautifiers**
**Boost it** Make the most of what you've got. Bronzer with shimmery, light-reflecting particles will boost your bust significantly. It'll make them 'pop' out and give them a youthful curve. Brush highlighter on each breast and blush in between them.

**Minimise it** You can minimise a big bust with v-necks (they divide and lengthen the torso); sweetheart necklines and wraparound cardigans; dark colours in matt fabrics on the top half; tailored shirts; curvy jackets nipped in at the waist; and coat dresses.

Make sure your bra fits you: if the band at the back rides up, you need one with a smaller back size; if the underwire is digging in under your armpit, your cups are too small; if you have indents where the straps have dug in then look for one smaller in the back and bigger in the cup; and if your breasts are falling through the bottom of the underwire, you need a bigger cup size.

# 31. Points on posture

**How you hold yourself can make you look and feel longer, leaner and more confident. Shoulders back now.**

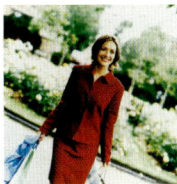

Forget balancing a few books on your head and walking elegantly around a room. These days improving posture is an altogether more athletic pursuit. The key to great posture is to stabilise your core, i.e. the muscles that run around your body – your natural corset if you like. Pilates is the ultimate tummy-flattening, posture-boosting discipline as it's based on firming precisely these muscles. Pilates can also be a great libido booster as strengthening your abs, back and pelvic floor can enhance sexual function and response.

## Here's an idea for you...

Been sitting down for too long? Counter bad posture with this exercise. Begin on all fours with your weight evenly distributed and your hands and knees shoulder-width apart. Pull your left knee towards your chest with your right hand, simultaneously curling your head towards your chest. Uncurl slowly, extending your left leg and right hand until they're horizontal to the floor; your back should be in a straight line. Repeat on the opposite side after placing your left knee and hand slightly forward of the starting position. Do five sequences; you should find you're moving across the floor.

## Stand tall

- Relax your shoulders down into your back. When they feel tight, raise them up to your ears, squeezing them up and together as hard as you can, as if you're doing an exaggerated shrug, then just drop them and feel the tension ease. Try squeezing your shoulder blades together behind you; it's a great way to keep your shoulders back.
- Make sure you put equal weight on each foot. If you're standing with more weight on one foot or with one foot turned out you'll look crooked.
- Keep your chin parallel to the floor.

## Sit up straight

- Sit at the end of your chair and slouch completely. Draw yourself up and accentuate the curve of your back as far as possible. Hold for a few seconds and then release the position slightly (about ten degrees). This is a good sitting posture.
- Make sure your back is straight and your shoulders back. Your buttocks should touch the back of your chair.

**Strengthen those abs**

Start on your hands and your knees. While exhaling raise your right arm and left leg until they're level with your torso. Keep your hips even and look down so that your neck is aligned. Contract your abs, but don't tuck your pelvis under or arch your back. Pull in your pelvic floor muscles and pull your tummy button in towards your backbone. Slowly return to the start and then repeat on the other side. Do two sets of eight repetitions on each side.

# 32. Sex up your legs

**How to slim, tone, smooth, soften and generally flatter them**

Nothing will produce more wolf whistles than a pair of slim, shapely legs. If you keep legs smooth, toned, bronzed and moisturised, they will take you a lot further in life than from A to B.

**Long and lean**

A combination of cardiovascular and resistance exercise is the best way to tone legs; aim for three thirty-minute cardio sessions such as running, rowing or cycling, and three sets of the exercises below per

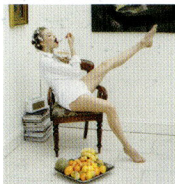

Here's an idea for you...

Be clever with tights. Black opaques make legs svelte and go with pretty much everything. Choose tights with vertical stripes to make your legs look longer and leaner. Fishnets can also look fantastic, but stick to more flattering narrow weaves and dark colours. Avoid red or white like the plague and don't team tights with minis unless you're a lady of the night.

week. These exercises can be done in the comfort of your home and will improve the muscular tone of your legs. Try the following exercises. Aim to do three sets of each exercise, three times a week.

**Thigh, bum and calf firmers**
*Straight leg lunge*
Stand on a step and then take a large stride off it, extending one leg back behind you. Your front knee should be over your front ankle and the back leg should be long with a slight bend at the knee. Keep the back knee and heel off the floor. Contract through your tummy muscles as you lift yourself back up to a straight position. Change legs. Do twelve on each leg, building up to three sets.

**Thigh toners**
*Squats*
Stand with your feet wider than hip-width apart, with your toes and knees pointing out at forty-five degrees and your hands on your thighs. Pull up through your tummy muscles. Bend your knees, lowering your torso towards the floor. Keep the weight on your heels, and your spine in neutral position with your tailbone pointing

down as you lower. Draw your weight onto one leg as you drag the other towards it. Use your inner thighs to draw your legs together. Draw your legs apart and repeat on the other side. Repeat twelve to fifteen times on each leg, again building up to three sets.

*Defining idea*

*'Darling, the legs aren't so beautiful, I just know what to do with them.'*
**MARLENE DIETRICH**

## Smooth and soft

For this you need to exfoliate regularly using a loofah, body brush or exfoliating mitt. Exfoliators are great for softening the hard skin on knees too. Keep legs well moisturised at all times; creams and lotions help plump up the upper layer of skin and make it look softer, smoother and younger.

## Bronzed and shimmery

A tan will automatically give the impression of longer, slimmer, more even-textured legs. Fake tan is the best way to get a safe year-round tan. Always exfoliate first and massage in a light moisturiser before applying your tanning product. Rubbing body oil into your legs will make them shimmer seductively.

# 33. Creating curves

**A dainty waist oozes sex appeal. Here's how to hone it, firm it and whittle it in weeks.**

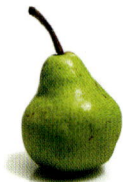

Studies show that waist to hip ratio – going in and out in all the right places – is a better gauge of a woman's attractiveness than the size of her breasts. Men of all cultures fancy women with small waists. To be precise, women with a 0.7 hip-to-waist ratio, i.e. waists that are 70% smaller than their hips. And that doesn't necessarily involve being thin! Think Sophia Loren and Marilyn Monroe.

The reason for this is biological. A small waist that curves into a generous hip equals fertility and youth – it's a sign that a woman has high levels of oestrogen and low levels of testosterone. In fact, in studies of IVF patients, women with a hip to waist ratio of more than 0.8 were less likely to conceive.

*Here's an idea for you...*

Invest in a gorgeous corset. Anything that boosts your bust and cinches your waist will do wonders for your rating in the bedroom.

Love handles won't simply disappear. You have to shed the fat first. Experts say that if your waist measures between 81 and 89 cm (32–35 inches), you're overweight. You need diet and exercising.

**Defining idea**

*'The curve is more powerful than the sword.'*
**MAE WEST**

## Waist-whittling exercises

*Twist crunches* Lie on your back with your knees bent, your feet flat on the floor and your fingers touching your ears. Contract your abdominal muscles and slowly lift your torso off the floor. When you can't lift any further, contract your side muscles and turn to the left. Then return your torso to the floor and repeat on the other side. Build up to three sets of ten on each side.

*The bridge* Adopt the press-up position, resting on your elbows. Pull your stomach muscles in tight towards your backbone, keeping your bottom down and your spine straight. Hold this position for as long as you can, being careful not to arch your back. To make it easier, drop to your knees. Keep looking down to the floor at all times. Build up to thirty seconds and repeat three to five times.

*Horizontal side support* Start by lying on your left side, resting on your left arm and with your legs extended outwards and your right foot on top of the left. Slowly lift your pelvis off the floor while supporting your weight on your left forearm and feet. Hold, keeping your other arm by your side, for ten to fifteen seconds without letting your pelvis drop down. Repeat five times on each side.

# 34. Chill out and lose weight

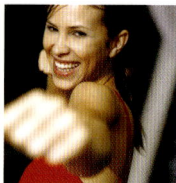

**Experts now say stress is related to weight gain. Which is why you need to beat stress, fast. The easiest way is by controlling what goes in your mouth.**

### Sugar balance

One thing you can do immediately is balance your blood sugar levels. Dense, fibrous foods such as lentils do this rather than sweet or starchy foods like gluey white loaves of bread or potatoes. Eat slow energy-releasing carbohydrates, or protein with slow energy-releasing carbohydrates, which will raise blood sugar levels slowly, improving your mood.

So, what effect does wildly fluctuating blood sugar levels have on mood? Well, in case your partner hasn't told you already, this can make you irritable,

*Here's an idea for you...*

Eat several snacks during the day rather than three great big meals. This will prevent too many massive peaks and dips in your blood sugar level so you'll be able to step off that blood sugar rollercoaster. Snack on apples, nuts and seeds – almonds and sunflower or pumpkin seeds are ideal. Or try oatcakes with goat's cheese, humous or cottage cheese. And if this doesn't appeal, fruit with yoghurt is always an option.

grouchy and fatigued. Not great
things to aspire to if you want to
handle your stress better.

*Defining idea*

'You are what you eat.'
**ANONYMOUS**

## Fat head

Omega-3 and omega-6 fats are called essential fats because they are.
Essential that is. Your body's hormones and your brain run on them
so make sure you're getting enough. Sources of omega-3 fats include
flax and hemp seeds, whereas omega-6 fats come from oily fish like
sardines, mackerel or salmon. And getting enough of the right sort
of fat has been shown to improve depression.

## Food and mood

An easy way to improve how you deal with stress is to reduce the
amount of tea and coffee you drink. These contain stimulants that
only make you more hyped up and tense. Try cutting down on those
lattes and see how you feel.

If you thought that tryptophan was a village in Wales, I'm afraid
you're wrong. Tryptophan is an amino acid (protein building block)
that can help raise levels of the mood-boosting neurotransmitter
serotonin. Foods high in tryptophan include figs, milk, tuna,
chicken, seaweed, sunflower seeds and yoghurt, but you need to
make sure you have plenty of B vitamins in place for your body to
process it (especially B3, B6, folic acid and biotin). You also need

vitamin C and zinc. Eating some slow energy-releasing carbohydrates with a tryptophan-rich food also helps your body process the tryptophan and turn it into serotonin.

# 35. Ready for a detox?

**Detox is such a big buzz word these days, but what exactly does it mean?**

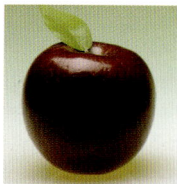

Basically it means cutting out rubbish – which of course means you'll lose weight, too. The big advantage is that you can tell yourself that you're improving your health – not dieting – and this is a powerful motivator if simply losing weight isn't enough for you. Taking stock of where you are is important because if you detox too quickly you could experience a number of unpleasant symptoms, such as headaches, lack of energy and generally feeling unwell. Don't think of doing a detox when you have an important week at work, as you might have a bit of a fuzzy head.

### Don't make me
Why should we put ourselves through a detox? Isn't it really hard work? Our bodies are in a constant state of renewal at cell level, but

if there's an overload of toxins either from food or environmental sources our bodies struggle to deal with them, effectively putting a strain on the kidneys and liver and taking away energy that could otherwise be used for living. A detox diet allows us to stop overloading the body with harmful substances and, if we give the body plenty of the right nutrients, it can speed up the elimination of toxins and promote cell renewal.

### Here's an idea for you...

Get a juicer and start making your own juice. You might like to try a combination of apple and blueberry or carrot and apple. Juices can be full of vitamins and minerals that help the detoxification systems important to the body. But remember to use organic fruit as there are pesticides on conventionally grown fruit.

**Warm-up**

If you're afraid of becoming Mr or Mrs Fuzzy Potatohead, then the thing to do is to start slowly over a period of one month. Choose in the first week to eliminate coffee, chocolate and caffeine drinks (cola drinks), replacing them with lots of water and herbal teas. In the second week, try eliminating wheat products (cakes, biscuits, pasta) and substitute them with rye bread or other grains such as brown rice, quinoa, buckwheat or millet. In the third week, try substituting dairy products for sheep and goat products. And in the fourth week, increase your water intake up to at least 2 litres (3.5 pints) of water a day, while avoiding alcohol.

You might want to take into consideration environmental toxins too and try to avoid them during this period. Are you a smoker? Do you regularly use aerosol sprays? Do you take lots of over-the-counter medication (for example, for headaches)? What about your exposure to traffic fumes? If you're a cyclist, consider wearing a mask to filter fumes.

# 36. Out there and doing it

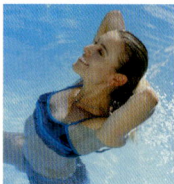

**Hate the gym? So, what are the alternatives?**

I hate the music in gyms. I hate the smell of them. I don't like the machines and they don't like me. I just don't think the gym is beautiful. No-one talks to each other because they're so busy doing exercise, there are all those mirrors, and it's so dehumanising – loud music, bright lights, functional, high speed. You're in and out of there with no connection to the rest of the human race. The other obvious thing wrong with the gym is that you join up and then don't go for a whole year, wasting huge sums of money.

## Getting it where you can

So, what other possibilities are
there? Go and exercise outside. You
don't have to be in the midst of the
glorious countryside for this one.
Your local park will do. Use the
park benches to stretch, use steps
to run up and use lamp-posts as
distance markers. Let your imagination run wild as to what you can
use in the environment to help you in your mission (no gym
fitness). Set goals – a good one might be to count the number of
times you run round the park, each time trying to improve upon
the last. I have a great little run that I do by the River Thames in
London (down by Chelsea Harbour) where you can see loads of
wildlife, cranes, fish, swans and ducks, despite being in the city.
What a pleasure.

Getting some aerobic exercise by running and walking will obviously
increase your cardiovascular fitness, and even in the city (away from
busy roads) you'll benefit from breathing 'fresh' air into your lungs.
Pumping your heart muscle is important to get your lymph system
moving – your lymph has no internal pump – and this helps banish
cellulite. Aerobic exercise is also thought to protect you against all sorts
of nasty diseases, including some types of cancers and heart disease,
plus it makes your bones stronger. So, get out there and do some
cardiovascular stuff. Run, jog or walk for at least 20 minutes each day.

### Here's an idea for you...

Exercising at home is another way to
avoid the gym. Why not check out
psychocalisthenics (www.pcals.com)?
This is a form of exercise that revitalises
your whole system yet takes just 15
minutes to do.

**Power walking** – Stride out when you walk. Get into it by loading your iPod up with some seriously good music.

**Jump higher** – Skipping is a wonderful way to get your ticker really going. Apparently, jumping rope has the calorie-burning capacity of jogging for one mile.

**Warm up and wind down** – Don't forget to stretch at the beginning and end of your workouts. Warm, stretched muscles are muscles that are less likely to be injured.

# 37. Have a heart (rate monitor)

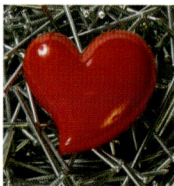

**Do you hate jogging/running? All that wobbly flesh jigging up and down?**

Tempted to throw away your running shoes and head straight back to the couch? Well, that's how I was until I had my Pauline conversion. You simply have to get a heart rate monitor. Now! No excuses. In my experience, this is the only way to get the running habit. You exercise according to your own fitness level and don't try to race ahead before you're ready. You could buy a heart rate monitor from www.polar.fi or www.heartratemonitor.co.uk or any good sports shop. Some gyms also sell them.

A heart rate monitor usually has two parts: a chest strap and a sports watch. The strap picks up your heartbeat, which is displayed on the watch. In this way you can tell if your training is too strenuous or not strenuous enough.

*Here's an idea for you...*

Try these two fabulous books that teach you how to exercise with heart rate monitors: *The Maffetone Method* by Dr Philip Maffetone and *Slow Burn* by Stu Mittleman. Also, if you really get into this you could get a monitor that allows you to set zones. An alarm will then sing out as soon as you stray from the selected zone. In other words, your watch will tick you off if you start to slack off or put your foot to the floor with a little too much gusto.

Don't go for the all-singing, all-dancing version of the heart rate monitor to start with. There are versions that will tell you how many calories you've burned, how far you've been on your training and record all sorts of things you might want to forget. If you're new to heart rate monitors then just buy a basic model like a Polar A3.

**Walk the walk**

Walking is a great way to get started. It's the safest work-out. We all know how to do it for starters! The intensity is low but it's great for burning fat. Just put on your heart rate monitor and a pair of trainers and hit the road. If you do decide to get into running in a serious way, you might consider an assessment with a physiotherapist who will let you know what type of stretching and other exercise would be good for you. A big one to watch out for is your knee health.

A heart rate monitor will:

- help you moderate your exercise intensity;
- help motivate you
- accurately measure your heart rate; and
- enable you to judge improvement over time, like having your own personal trainer.

# 38. Gotta run

**Run for your health, social life, waistline or sanity. There are as many reasons to run as there are runners.**

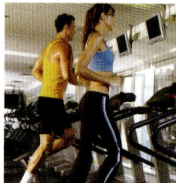

Never mind your style or speed, the fact remains that as bipeds we were pretty much made for this running malarkey. It's relatively cheap (though you should look to spend as much as you can afford on decent shoes and a good sports bra) and anyone can do it pretty much anywhere (though with greater and lesser degrees of pleasure). It's still about the best calorie-burning exercise known to man and it builds up bone density, endurance, toned thighs and stronger heart and lungs. More than that though, for many of us it can be a special time, a quiet time set aside for thinking things over or perhaps not thinking things over. Most runners also talk about feelings of enhanced self-esteem, so what's holding you back?

*Here's an idea for you...*

Having a running partner can make all the difference. It can make time fly as you chat and it can help motivate you to show up in the first place. Look online and in local papers for running clubs.

For many, it's the fear that we just can't do it. So, take it one step at a time (so to speak). I know a man called Luke Cunningham who found he wasn't so keen on what he saw in the mirror and decided to try jogging. He started by running for a few minutes, stopping to catch his breath and then running back. And he still talks of the sense of satisfaction from running over seven minutes each way – a full quarter of an hour of running. Luke now competes in seven-day events over hundreds of kilometres of desert.

Just take it at your own pace and plan where you will run. Take enough money to buy a bus ticket back in case you get tired or sprain something. Know where you are going and where you will find water, such as a drinking fountain, a café or from a bottle you take with you. Try not to have to cross roads (it's easy for your attention to wander at crucial moments) or run past potential stress

factors such as a corner where the
local kids hang out or where
there's a territorial aggressive dog.
Don't forget to think about the
weather – runners suffer sunburn
too and if there's any wind it's
always easier to set out against the
wind and run back with it behind
you.

# 39. Gym bunny

**The gym can prove to be extremely
effective and convenient in terms of your
fitness goals and it doesn't have to be
boring**

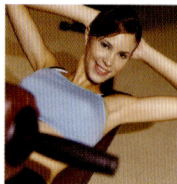

Remember that your ultimate reward is looking and feeling
sensational. Most gyms have classes ranging from yoga, Pilates, kickboxing and circuit training to dance classes, spinning (a work-out on
a stationary bike), and running and rowing clubs. Find some classes
that suit you, and then simply enjoy them! Find a gym that you'll

actually go to in order to keep excuses like it not being on your way to/from work at bay.

### Include weight-training

Weight training doesn't mean you'll end up looking like Arnie. It's a great way to add tone and definition to your body and will increase lean muscle mass, thus help to manage weight. Using weights has the added bonus of strengthening your bones. Change your technique from time to time.

Try these:

- **Circuit training** This can be done in a class or you can make up your own. Keep moving from machine to machine and include free-weights and some abdominal work.
- **Core stability** A very important factor in overall strength, this engages the stabilising muscles and initially may feel like you're not working very hard. Take part in a class or have a trainer show you how to use the gym balls. Building up core stability can help prevent injuries and improve posture. It's a departure from just giving it welly on all the machines.

*Here's an idea for you...*

Get the right kit. You'll feel like you're taking the whole thing seriously and having spent the money you'll have to turn up! Supportive, breathable shoes are a must. Wear an outfit that you'll be comfortable in. But ensure that whatever you choose allows for a good range of movement. Women: ensure that your bra offers good support for your chosen activity. See www.lessbounce.com.

## Defining idea

*'The worst moment in life is the moment you lose faith in your dreams. Never let it happen.'*
**MICHAEL COLGAN, specialist in the field of optimum nutrition for US Olympic sports people**

And above all:

- **Focus!** Don't just plonk yourself on the exercise bike with your favourite weekly. Find out with the help of a trainer what your ideal training zone is.
- **Drink!** A lack of water can affect your strength, stamina and ability to burn fat.
- **Rest!** There is such a thing as overtraining. As you become fitter you may be able to train longer and harder, but muscles need rest to repair, recover and strengthen. Overtraining can deplete the immune system as well as your mood and energy levels.
- **Ouch!** If you feel pain, especially sustained pain, see someone about it – gym staff are the first port of call. Pain is the body's way of telling you something is wrong, so don't ignore it.

# 40. Stretching the point

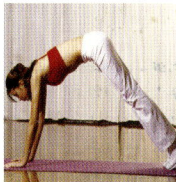

**Stretching achieves long, lean muscles – people who stretch look slimmer and walk taller**

Fail to stretch and you'll be stiff and end up walking like John Wayne. Not a good look...

*Maintenance stretch* At the end of your exercise hold the stretch for 10 to 15 seconds or so. Remember to stretch all of the muscles you're using.

**Common stretches**

Take time to find out about the stretches specific to your sport and then take the time to do them. The most common stretches are:

*Quadriceps* While standing upright, balance on one leg and bend the other so you can catch your foot in your hand. Flex your foot gently

## Here's an idea for you...

If you like the idea of developmental stretching and would like to be suppler, try Bikram yoga. Sessions are conducted in a steamy room to keep muscle temperatures high and help suppleness. There's only one set of moves so it's easy to learn but takes forever to master. The emphasis is on developing the range of movement and stretch in joints and muscles.

Defining idea

*'When you engage in systematic, purposeful action, using and stretching your abilities to the maximum, you cannot help but feel positive and confident about yourself.'*
**BRIAN TRACY, US author and motivational speaker**

back up to your buttocks and don't worry about putting a hand out on a wall or partner to keep your balance. Very slightly bend the knee of the leg you're balancing on and tip the hips forward to feel the stretch down the front of your thigh. Hold. Gently go back to standing and switch legs.

*Calves* Stand four or five steps away from and facing a wall. Keep your left foot in its original position but place your right foot halfway between you and the wall. Reach forward with your outstretched arms so you're leaning against the wall with them. Your right leg should now be bent and your left leg straight out behind you with the sole of the foot flat on the floor. Feel the stretch up the back of the calf. Hold, then gently go back to standing and switch legs.

*Triceps* Reach one arm straight up above your head then bend it at the elbow so your hand is now behind your neck. Reach up with the other hand, take the first elbow, and gently pull it down and across in the direction of the pulling arm's shoulder. Hold, release, switch.

*Shoulder* Hold your arm out straight in front of you then move it across your body placing the other hand on the upper arm between elbow and shoulder. Use that hand to push the arm in towards the chest. Hold, release, switch.

# 41. The Hoover work-out

**Why not make a real difference to your fitness by grabbing all the everyday opportunities?**

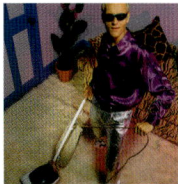

The gym is great, but the exercise you'll stick at is the kind built into your day. Here's a really good life tip from a London cabby I spoke to last week:

The cabby had a fifteen-stone wife until she decided to go for a walk with her friend three times a week. Each session lasted for an hour. It wasn't a pushing-it-walk mind, but a little bit more than a stroll. She'd piled on the pounds since having her two children and had tried every diet under the sun. So, she decided to give up the diets, eat a wee bit more sensibly and take up walking. Five months later and she is just under ten stone, without doing anything more complicated than going for a walk down by the river where she lives. She finds that walking is a great de-stressor too and manages to combine it with a gossip with her friend. She also loves the peace and quiet away from the kids, which she dumps on her hubby for an hour, scooting out the door with a cheery wave.

Depending on where you live and work, a great way to carve the time out is to walk to work. As you won't really get sweaty, you won't have to worry about shower facilities as you might following a session down the gym. I carry a clean top in my rucksack and put my wallet, keys and 'handbag' stuff in there too. Put on a good pair of gym shoes, put your smart work ones in the rucksack, and off you go.

**Strut your funky stuff!**

Find everyday excuses for exercise at home too. I put on Meat Loaf's *Bat out of Hell*, get the Hoover out and wiggle my stuff about in that dust. And no doubt you've heard it before but walk the escalators, walk up stairs, don't take the lift. Thin, lithe folk are always in motion – be like them. We're designed to be in continuous movement.

# 42. Take a walk on the wild side

**Take your walk to the next level**

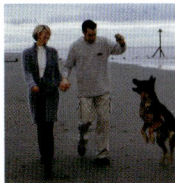

Be more adventurous in your walk – you could get hooked. Walking can mean more than popping out to the corner shop for twenty Marlboro. Why not take a chance on adventure walking? Even if you only plan a walking weekend every so often – a special weekend in the country once or twice a year – it will inspire you for the smaller everyday stuff like getting out to the park or walking to work. Make sure you're kitted out with the right gear before you set out.

Great wet-weather gear is a must. I'm not talking fisherman's yellow galoshes and capes –these days you can get very light wet-weather gear that will fold up and fit into your pocket. Don't just get the top, invest in the trousers as well, as there's nothing worse than being in the middle of nowhere with wet, cold and soggy trousers and no chance of changing them for the next 50 miles. There's no such thing as bad weather just inappropriate gear!

The second vital bit of kit for your proper walking experience is the right boots. Remember that you could well have thick socks to allow for so don't buy them too small. Talking of socks, it's worth getting proper walking socks. A good outdoor shop should be able to advise you on the right kind of boots and socks for you. The boots need to be protective of the ankles, waterproof and not too heavy. They also need a good grip – the proper lace-up ones are ideal (check out www.snowandrock.com).

Defining idea

'You cannot teach a crab to walk in a straight line.'
**ARISTOPHENES**

The other essential piece of kit is your rucksack or daypack. Choose one with a middle strap that goes round your tummy as this will help to protect your back. These days there are rucksacks that make sure that the material isn't next to your back so you don't get too sweaty carrying it. Make sure you get one with loads of pockets for maps, bits of string, etc. Also, pack a whistle just in case you need to attract attention. And a hat, good sunglasses and some sunscreen. A map is always a good idea, as long as you can read it! And you'll need to carry at least a litre of water. Obviously in boiling temperatures you'll need more. Don't forget to pack a small medical kit that includes some rehydration sachets (electrolyte formulas) and some plasters for those pesky blisters.

# 43. Instant miracle-workers

**How to perfect your posture**

Perfect posture could be your short-cut to a leaner, longer shape. You'll be breathing better too. Try this: Sit up straight for five minutes with your head up and shoulders dropped. Concentrate on your breathing. How do you feel? Relaxed? Of course you do! So, where can you take it next?

## Pilates

Pilates seems to be the new buzz word, although Joseph H. Pilates actually perfected his programme in the US in the 1920s. Pilates is a re-education programme for your muscles, which are used to a lifetime of abuse. One of the major features of Pilates is core stability

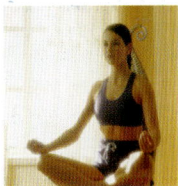

## Here's an idea for you...

Experiment with different methods by getting DVDs of your new fads. If you enjoy doing a particular discipline in the comfort of your own home take a course of classes where you start right from the beginning and master the basics – it can be very demotivating if everyone is better than you, despite the fact that most posture disciplines profess not to be competitive.

and strength. A teacher is best to take you though the basics of Pilates or you can end up wondering whether you're getting it right. Most gyms offer Pilates – take advantage of their classes because one-to-one Pilates tuition can be expensive.

### Alexander Technique

Think how easily small kids move. However, as we grow older and tense ourselves up against the worries of the world our posture suffers, often with disastrous results such as migraine, arthritis, neck pain and back pain. Many postural problems have stemmed from over-tensed neck muscles, which interfere with how the head relates to the spine. The Alexander Technique is often taught using verbal instruction and the physical guidance of a teacher's correcting hands. It's often taught privately so prepare yourself for an investment. Check out www.alexandertechnique.com, a comprehensive source of information.

## Just be with T'ai chi

T'ai chi is a slow-moving
choreography and is considered a
martial art – each minute
movement shifts the body's weight
subtly from one leg to the other
throughout the whole routine. Moment to moment attention is
required at all times, thus t'ai chi is a type of meditation through
movement. Practised properly, flexibility, balance and strength are
all within your grasp. Look for t'ai chi advertised locally. Again, many
gyms now run classes.

*Defining* idea

'Never grow a wishbone, daughter,
where your backbone ought to be.'
**CLEMENTINE PADDLEFORD, author**

## Back problems?

What about getting a chiropractor, osteopath or physiotherapist to
check your posture out and help fix it? A chiropractor is really
concerned about your spine; osteopathic treatment concentrates on
the relationship between the structures of the body – the skeleton,
muscles, ligaments and connective tissues – and relieving muscle
tension is often a big part of the therapy; and physiotherapists can
assess your posture but often make *you* do the work by giving you
exercises to do at home.

# 44. Get on yer bike

**It's difficult to injure yourself cycling because it's such a low-impact form of exercise**

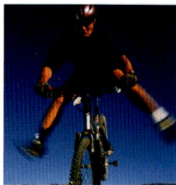

Cycling will also burn off extra fat and reduce stress, plus it's a great way to tone your legs and the nicest way to see the countryside.

Here's an idea for you...

If cycling gets your wheels turning consider combining it with a holiday. Find a company that'll give you an itinerary suited to your energy level plus accompanying cars to drop off your baggage at the next hotel on the route, then all you'll have to do is pedal and enjoy the view.

**Stretch it out**

Some cyclists, particularly those of you who hop on your bikes and cycle to work, rarely bother to warm up. If this is you, you might want to take a long hard look at your flexibility and posture. The main thigh muscle (the rectus femoris) has a high chance of being damaged unless you stretch it out properly. Another thing to watch out for is tight hamstrings and pulled hip flexors (at the top of the front of the thigh), which can happen often if you don't take time to stretch. A heel dig stretch might help as a basic exercise to help all three of these common muscle problems. Simply lift your toes, keeping your knee straight and your heel on the ground, until you feel a pull in

the back and front of the calf and
upper thigh.

Hunching at the handlebars can
lead to a permanent rounding of
the shoulders and back. A typical yoga exercise can help counteract
this – the Cobra. Lie on your front with your arms by your sides and
lift your chest and head until you feel the movement in your back
and shoulders.

## Getting the right bike for you

Mountain bikes are rarely suitable for riding in town and that goes
for racing bikes too, however flash they may look. Having your head
down when you ride is a sure way of going headlong into a bus! If
you've splashed out on a new bike, consider getting it sprayed with
nasty black paint in order to stop other people thinking what a
beautiful new bike you have and stealing it.

Swallow saddles (www.brooksengland.com) are back in vogue. These
are long pointy saddles with an unfeasibly small sitting area that
must owe more to aesthetics than to comfort as I imagine it's akin
to sitting on a knife. I recommend looking at a seat that has a three-
layered saddle of gel/foam/elastic that reduces pressure on the
prostate and pubic bones (www.lookin.it). Aaah, that's more like it!

# 45. Yoga

**Yoga is about being rather than doing. It's non-competitive and a great balancer for the type of exercise you might do at the gym.**

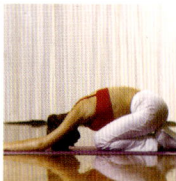

Not so long ago, if you admitted you did yoga you'd have been classed as a New Age weirdo and given a wide berth. Today, if you're not into yoga you're the weird one. More to the point, have you ever seen a fat yoga devotee? So, get with the programme!

Although yoga has evolved to incorporate quite a few different types, you're missing the point if you're using yoga to 'get a work-out'. Check out www.yogapoint.com for a guide to all the different types of yoga and pick the one that sounds interesting for you. You might want to experiment with the different types by going to a few classes. Or ask around, as friends might be able to give you advice.

*Here's an idea for you…*

As an alternative to hiring a private teacher, which can be quite expensive, club together with a couple of friends for some really worthwhile tuition in a small group once a week. You can always go to classes at the gym the rest of the time.

In essence though, all types of yoga are about using the body and breathing to help calm the mind in order to produce a feeling of wellbeing. Yoga is a great stress buster if ever there was one and it's easy to do at any age so it's never too late to start. Flexibility is a vital component, both physically and mentally – a flexible mind equals a flexible body. Yoga generally uses asanas (postures) that usually retain their ancient names: the fish, the bridge, the bow, the scorpion, etc. They are believed to bring benefits to different areas of the body and are held for a period of time to stretch and strengthen muscles. The shoulder-stand asana, for example, is said to massage the thyroid and bring benefits to the mind through improving blood circulation to the head. Worth a try? The simplest asana is the corpse position, which involves lying down on your back on the floor with your eyes closed. Your breathing should be slow and steady, and your arms should be held at a 45-degree angle away from the body.

Yoga is really a lifestyle rather than simply an exercise discipline. It incorporates 'proper' breathing or relaxation and a 'proper' diet. It's powerful stuff that's deceptively simple and amazingly dynamic. A proper diet, according to the yogis, is usually a vegetarian diet comprising Sattic foods such as wholemeal grains and fresh fruit and vegetables. It would be hard not to lose weight on a diet like this, wouldn't it?

*Defining idea*

'*The soul that moves in the world of senses in harmony...finds rest in quietness.*'
**BHAGAVAD GITA**

111

# 46. Team spirit

**If you left sports and team games behind with teenage crushes, acne and underage drinking, then perhaps you're missing out**

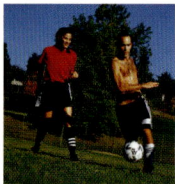

*Here's an idea for you...*

Consider the likes of roller hockey, fencing and Gaelic games, as sports that are completely different from anything you did when younger won't come with any historical baggage, including preconceived ideas about whether or not it matters to be good at it.

Games are often more fun when you're a grown-up. As an adult you have the option of taking up a sport simply for the pleasure of it. If you take up a new game now, you don't have to be good at it, you simply have to enjoy it. You'll find a club at your level for most adult team games, and it's likely to be one that will be profoundly grateful that you show up at all. In return, you'll get a chance to break out of your old routine and be more active. Sports aren't just about fitness either. For many, sport is a means of making new friends or getting away from their normal lives.

## Racquet games

For many of us the idea of playing a sport leads directly to thoughts of tennis or squash, which is great except that almost all racquet games are sprint sports that require skill, stamina and explosive strength. They can be great fun and they have a social world all of their own, but to get the most out of them you really need to get fit to play them, rather than play them to get fit. Have you ever considered badminton? Although it can be a very fast game, it's about the only racquet game that can truly be played leisurely between like-minded people.

Defining idea

'Any kind of exercise is generally better than no exercise at all. Walking is better for you than sitting in front of a television set and playing a sport is better for your health than just being a spectator.'
**ARNOLD SCHWARZENEGGER**

**Ball games**

Ball games like football (soccer) or rugby are also sprint sports where walking and jogging alternate with sprinting. Instead of going straight for the main game, you may find there's more knockabout fun to be had from smaller versions of the sport like five-a-side footie or seven-a-side rugby.

**Bowling**

Bowling isn't the world's most active activity, but it's social and gets you active. Lawn bowling has a more sedate image, though the skills aren't dissimilar from its more youthful ten-pin cousin, and the French game of boules can now be seen on beaches and in local clubs around the planet. The great thing about something like ten-pin bowling is that anyone can have a go and the kit you need (bowls and bowling shoes) will be provided by the bowling hall.

# 47. Home spa

**Pampering yourself at home will spur on your weight loss.**

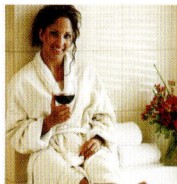

### Wake up you lemon!

First things first, hop out of bed and go and make yourself a cup of hot water with lemon or lime. This will help support your liver in its cleansing process. You might also decide that a delicious smoothie is in order for a delicious, vitalising breakfast.

Before your bathing rituals, start your morning with a skin-brushing session. As well as keeping the inside in, the skin is an important organ of elimination. Dry skin brushing is a great but inexpensive way to boost blood and lymphatic circulation and remove dead skin cells. Lymphatic fluid brings nutrients to cells and carries away toxins, but isn't pumped by the heart, instead it is moved primarily by movement and massage. The skin may feel a little tender at first, but by jove it's worth it because when you have your cold shower, your skin will tingle all over. Actually, you might want to start with a tepid shower – I won't call you a coward. Remember, you have to suffer to be beautiful and this is helping with the cellulite – so get on with it! Choose a natural bristle brush with a long handle, start at

Defining idea

*'Beauty is only skin deep.'*
**A traditional saying, but who cares?**

114

the feet and brush upwards towards the heart in long sweeping figure-of-eight movements. For your arm and chest you are brushing down towards the heart – don't brush any really sensitive bits!

Smell is very important and aromatherapy oils can either be added to yet another bathing experience or added to a little water in a special oil burner and heated gently by a nightlight candle. Be careful though as essential oils are highly flammable. You can get your oils from www.tisserand.com.

Treat yourself to a detox clay wrap. Shape Changers (www.shapechangers.co.uk) are a favourite and contain 100% clay with a range of aromatherapy oils. They're designed to cleanse and tone the skin and draw out toxins – check out the inch-loss potential on this one!

In the afternoon go to your local gym for a sauna or a steam and, if you're not sick of the whole detox experience, before you go to bed strap on two detox plasters (www.koyotakara.com) to the soles of your feet. When you wake the next morning, you'll be horrified to find brown gunky stuff on the plaster, which is your own personal toxin dump.

*Here's an idea for you...*

Hang a muslin bag or old sock (a clean one please) filled with porridge oats under the hot tap while running your bath. Oats contain properties that are very soothing and moisturising to the skin, especially for those who suffer with dry skin conditions such as eczema. Don't let the porridge fall into the water, as this would be very messy.

# 48. Use your imagination

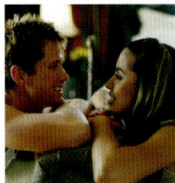

**Consider this the instruction manual for your most powerful and under-utilised tool you possess. Your brain.**

Harness you mind and weight loss is easy. In the West we try to protect ourselves against life by using logic. We put great emphasis on school subjects like maths, English, science and languages, and imagination and creativity are effectively banned by the age of five. Can anyone remember the shock of going from pre-school to junior school and realising that dipping your hands in paint and scribbling on huge pieces of paper wasn't what was expected from you anymore?

Defining idea

*'Imagination is more important than knowledge.'*
**ALBERT EINSTEIN**

We totally over-exercise this logical (left) side of the brain to the massive detriment of our creative (right) side, which is also responsible for intuition. Before dismissing this idea as childish, take note that many of the world's great sportsmen are using this technique, which first became popular with the 'Inner Game' books. A proven way to improve your game is to use your imagination to play the shot in your head first, practice in your inner gym and then actually do it in reality. Performance will increase dramatically. The opposite too is true. If you 'see' yourself failing, you will.

If you could start rehearsing your life in your head, would your 'game' of life improve? Certainly the reverse is true. Bridget Jones' vision of ending up as a lonely old lady devoured by dogs will only come true if that's what you focus on. It's the classic case of the self-fulfilling prophecy.

### Here's an idea for you...

Start by programming your day. Sit in a chair, close your eyes and visualise how your day is going to be. Remember, this isn't based on reality but only held back by the confines of your imagination. For example, visualise leaving the house, the pleasant walk to the station, the receptionist's smile or the warm greeting of your spouse on returning home. See if you get a better day by imagining one. This works best when you're going to give a presentation or make an important deal. Practising for an event like this will hone your performance and knock the edge of your nerves.

If you doubt the power of imagination over your ability to perform, just think about this. If I was to offer £1,000 to anyone prepared to walk a 2-metre plank of wood that I'd placed on the floor, there would be a line of people queuing round the block. Yet if I was to place the same plank 100 metres above ground between two buildings, those same people would be phoning the funny farm to have me taken away. Imagine yourself succeeding at your healthy eating regime. Imagine yourself walking into a room and everyone being stunned at how you look. Imagine shopping for clothes – and see vividly – that label a dress size smaller. Imagine yourself, in glorious technicolor – SLIM!

# 49. It's all about You

**The worm has turned! Now it's time to put yourself first**

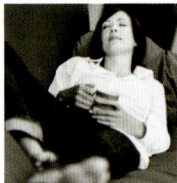

If you're not looking after yourself you're in no position to look after others. And it's only by making time for yourself that you can achieve your goals. The first place to start in terms of putting yourself first is to establish where your own personal boundaries lie. Knowing your boundaries is being able to say 'No' because you know what you want and which direction you're heading in your life. Saying 'No' is an art form, but you don't have to suddenly become Mr or Mrs Horrible. The trick is not to volunteer in the first place.

Another trick that will both carve yourself time and make yourself the most important person in your life is to schedule. Put your time down in your diary and stick to it. Your diary should consist of appointments that you have to do at a certain time (e.g. your weekly sales meeting), appointments that don't have to be done at a specific time (e.g. the meeting with the personnel manager to talk over various staffing issues) and appointments that don't have to be done at any specific time. That's where you start scheduling. Put your holidays in your diary *now*. Put down the trip to the beach *now*. The same goes with your son's nativity play or your gym sessions. Prioritise yourself *now*. And if, for instance, you book in half a day's holiday to go to your wife's graduation and the sales director for the whole of the world market rings and asks if you can have a meeting that afternoon say, 'No, but I could make Friday morning.' 'Fine,' he'll reply. It really is that simple, you just have to hold your nerve.

And why is this so important? Because you'll also start scheduling exercise sessions and not get diverted. You'll have more energy and enthusiasm for what's important to you. And you'll no longer comfort eat because you'll be in control of your life.

## Here's an idea for you...

Book out an entire day to do exactly what you want (within the boundaries of the law, obviously). Plan your day meticulously, as if you're doing it for someone else. What would you like to do? Go to an art gallery? Check into a health spa for the day? Go to the zoo? Have a long bath then go to bed with a good book? Make space for yourself in your life. You need this space to be yourself, to be creative, to be regenerated. Don't feel guilty about it. Enjoy!

## Defining idea

'*I want to be alone!*'
**GRETA GARBO**

# 50. Scoop!

**Pilates is all about getting the pelvic floor and transversus muscles into play**

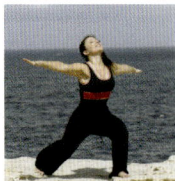

The real secret to a toned tum is a taut transversus. Activate those deep internal muscles to improve your posture and, yes, look better in that bathing suit. For that to happen, you gotta learn to 'scoop'. If we're told to pull in our stomachs, we do so from the front of our stomachs, trying to squeeze in rather than tense from the inside out. But to activate the transversus that's what we have to do.

## Here's an idea for you...

When you're working on your Pilates exercises in the privacy of your own home, take the soft belt out of your dressing gown or towelling bath robe and just knot it loosely around your hips so it's on the B-line. Now do your Pilates routine and let the belt remind you to constantly tauten up from below the navel. Make sure it's a soft belt, loosely knotted. Try this with a belt with buckle and notches and you run the risk of doing yourself a mischief.

First, stand straight, and pull in your stomach. Now try this:

Stand in neutral as before, feet hip-width apart, relaxed but not slumped. Draw a line with your fingers from one hip to the other across your tum. That's what Pilates instructors call the 'B-Line'. Find the centre of that line ('B' marks the spot), it should be a couple of inches below your navel.

Rest your finger on that spot and now try to pull the stomach in again but from that spot. Feel different? Feel as if you're working different muscles? Well you should be, and if you're contracting

*Defining idea*

'He who does not mind his belly, will hardly mind anything else.'
**SAMUEL JOHNSON**

from that point, then you should be working the transversus. The trick is to remember that however much you're trying to pull navel to spine, the way to bring your backbone and bellybutton together is not to focus on the navel at all, but rather on a point a couple of inches below it.

## The scoop/zipping up

When instructors talk about 'scooping' or 'zipping up' they're referring to the same thing. The idea is not to hollow out your stomach by pulling in the front, but instead to start right deep in the pelvis and tighten up from there. Zipping is a visualisation technique to help you get there. Instead of sucking in that stomach, imagine instead that there's a zip running from the pelvic floor up to the ribs. Start to zip up from the very bottom and you should engage the pelvic muscles and the transversus rather than the abdominis. Do this regularly and you'll tighten your tum. Throw in a few Pilates classes too and you'll soon be sporting that crop-top with pride.

# 51. Post Office Pilates

**Pilates is brilliant for toning you up fast – here you learn how to play the waiting game to win.**

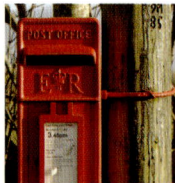

You will spend five years of your life standing in line. In Britain queuing is the unofficial national sport. It's being proposed as a relay event to the Olympic Committee and the discipline of First-day-of-the-sales Full Contact Queuing may soon be recognised as a formal martial art. In the meantime you might as well use some of that time on your feet to keep your body on its toes, as it were.

*Here's an idea for you...*

Lightly place the tips of your fingers between your navel and your knickers as you breathe. Feel the navel being pulled in and the tautness of your abdominal muscles as they rise and fall with the incoming breath.

It doesn't matter if you're standing in line for stamps, waiting for a bus or queuing for the border at Burkina Faso, you can always use the time to tone your torso.

First make sure you're standing with your feet hip-width apart, facing directly forward, knees very slightly bent and your shoulders nice and relaxed but not slumped. Tilt your pelvis forwards and backwards until you find the midpoint. If you genuinely are in line for an immigration official, police checkpoint or anything at all when in prison, then it's best not to rock your pelvis forward and back too vigorously. You might be sending out the wrong signals. Without bending your neck forwards, tilt your head so that your chin drops very slightly forward to extend the neck and help elongate the spine.

Breathe deeply. Really deeply, right down into your lower abdomen. Time to contemplate your navel. Focusing on your belly button, use your abdominal muscles to pull it right in towards your spine and up towards your ribs. Keep breathing in deep into the abdomen – it may seem a little strange at first but you should be able to do this without relaxing your stomach muscles. The aim is not to have your stomach clenched like a fist, but instead taut and elastic so that it is flattened but still rises as you draw air into your body.

Now breathe into your stomach, and gently out again for ten long, slow breaths. Of course you don't actually breathe into your stomach, but that's how it should feel. Concentrate on that stomach, on keeping your shoulders relaxed, and on emptying all the air out of your lungs as you breathe out.

Hey presto – stress relief and tummy toning all in one.

# 52 . Stuck on those last 7 lb?

**That stubborn half a stone is hard to shift whether you are near the end of your weight loss programme or that 7 lb is all you want to lose to begin with**

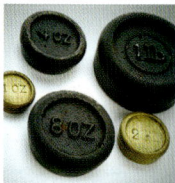

### Defining idea

*'It's OK to let yourself go, just as long as you let yourself back.'*
**MICK JAGGER**

It's such a small amount, you'd think it would pack its bags and leave without a whimper. But no, that half a stone always seems to be trickiest to shift. Here are five ways to push to the end.

1. How consistent are you? There are some experts who say as long as you eat sensibly for 80% of the time, you can relax a little for the other 20%. This could translate as making the healthiest choices all week and then eating whatever you like at the weekend. However, there's a big difference between relaxing a little and having a total blow-out every weekend. If you opt for the blow-outs, your week's calorie intake will stack up and your healthful efforts will be for nothing. That dull word 'moderation' springs to mind, but it really is a good concept to live by.

2. A simple way to cut a few calories is to cut out carbohydrates with your evening meal. You could try it every night for a couple of weeks, or every other night if that's more convenient. As long as your other meals and snacks are nutrionally balanced with some carbohydrate, you won't be missing out and you'll definitely see a difference on the scales.

3. Spice up your life with a few hot peppers in your lunch or dinner. Pepper eaters have less of an appetite and feel full quicker, according to Canadian research. The compound capsaicin that is found in peppers temporarily speeds your metabolism.

4. Include calcium in your diet, as, along with other substances in dairy foods, it seems to help your body burn excess fat faster. In a 2003 study, women who ate low fat yoghurt and cheese and drank low fat milk three or four times in a day lost 70% more body fat than women who didn't eat dairy at all.

5. Don't eat when you're not hungry. It seems obvious, but think about it next time you put food in your mouth. Ask yourself 'Am I really hungry?' before that second mouthful.

### Here's an idea for you...

Variety may be the spice of life, but too many choices can make you eat more. Research has shown that volunteers ate 44% more than a control group when offered a variety of dishes rather than the same amount of one dish. Similarly a group offered six flavours of jelly beans in one bowl ate nearly 70% more than those offered the same flavours in separate bowls – so even perception of variety seems to count too!

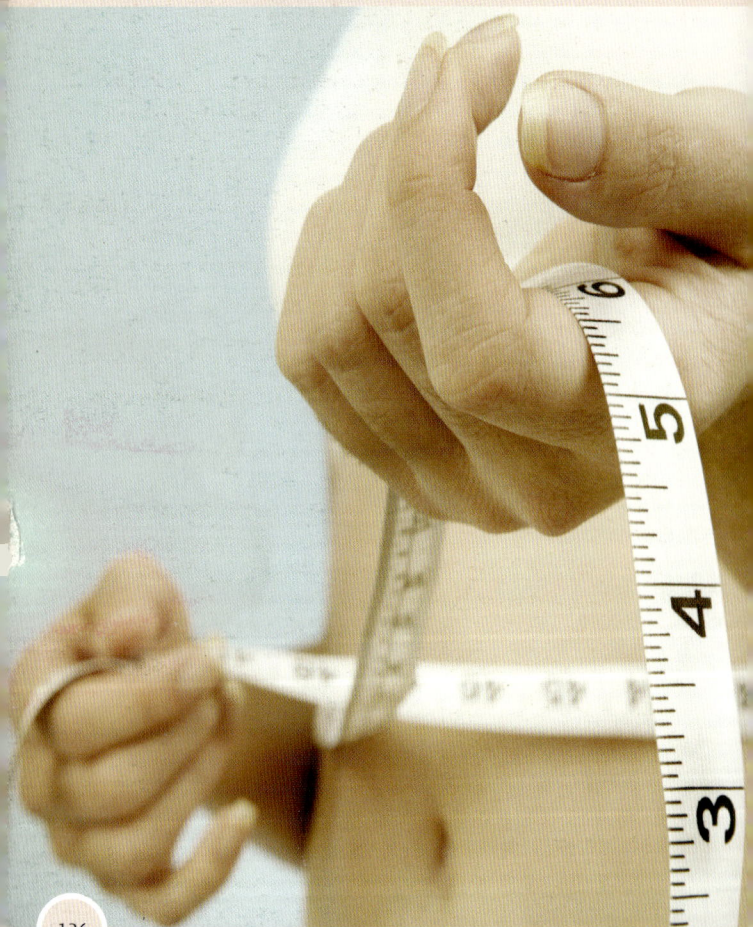

**52**
brilliant ideas

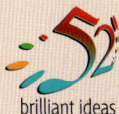

*Drop a dress size: 52 brilliant little ideas to lose weight and stay slim* is published by Infinite Ideas, creators of the acclaimed 52 Brilliant Ideas series. If you found this book helpful, you may want to take advantage of this special offer exclusive to all readers of *Drop a dress size*. Choose any two books from the selection below and you'll get one of them free of charge*. See overleaf for prices and details on how to place your order.

- **Be incredibly sexy:** 52 brilliant ideas for sizzling sensuality
- **Cellulite solutions:** 52 brilliant ideas for super smooth skin
- **Healthy cooking for kids:** 52 brilliant ideas to dump the junk
- **Inspired creative writing:** 52 brilliant ideas from the master wordsmiths
- **Look gorgeous always:** 52 brilliant ideas to find it, fake it and flaunt it
- **Stress proof your life:** 52 brilliant ideas for taking control
- **Upgrade your brain:** 52 brilliant ideas for everyday genius
- **Win at the gym:** Secrets of fitness and health success

For more detailed information on these books and others published by Infinite Ideas please visit www.infideas.com

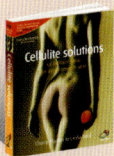

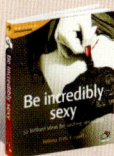

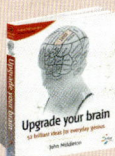

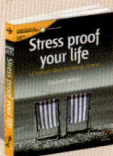

*Postage at £2.75 per delivery address is additional.

Choose any two titles from below and receive one of them free.

| Qty | Title | RRP |
|-----|-------|-----|
|  | Be incredibly sexy | £12.99 |
|  | Cellulite solutions | £12.99 |
|  | Healthy cooking for kids | £12.99 |
|  | Inspired creative writing | £12.99 |
|  | Look gorgeous always | £12.99 |
|  | Stress proof your life | £12.99 |
|  | Upgrade your brain | £12.99 |
|  | Win at the gym | £12.99 |
|  | Subtract £12.99 if ordering two titles |  |
|  | Add £2.75 postage per delivery address |  |
|  | **Final TOTAL** |  |

Name: ..............................................................................................

Delivery address: .............................................................................

..............................................................................................................

..............................................................................................................

E-mail:............................Tel (in case of problems): ...........................

**By post** Fill in all relevant details, cut out or copy this page and send along with a cheque made payable to Infinite Ideas. Send to: Drop a dress size BOGOF, Infinite Ideas, 36 St Giles, Oxford OX1 3LD. **Credit card orders over the telephone** Call +44 (0) 1865 514 888. Lines are open 9am to 5pm Monday to Friday. Just mention the promotion code 'DADSAD06.'

Please note that no payment will be processed until your order has been dispatched. Goods are dispatched through Royal Mail within 14 working days, when in stock. We never forward personal details on to third parties or bombard you with junk mail. This offer is valid for UK and RoI residents only. Any questions or comments please contact us on 01865 514 888 or email info@infideas.com.